D0563915

Healthy Eating for Life
for Children

PHYSICIANS COMMITTEE FOR
RESPONSIBLE MEDICINE

John Wiley & Sons, Inc.

Menus and recipes by Jennifer Raymond

Published by John Wiley & Sons, Inc., New York
Published simultaneously in Canada

Design and production by Navta Associates, Inc.

This publication is designed to provide accurate and authoritative information in regard to the subject matter covered. It is sold with the understanding that the publisher is not engaged in rendering professional services. If professional advice or other expert assistance is required, the services of a competent professional person should be sought.

Library of Congress Cataloging-in-Publication Data:

Healthy eating for life for children / Physicians Committee for Responsible Medicine.
    p. cm.
   Includes index.
   ISBN 0-471-43621-6 (pbk.)
   1. Eating disorders in children. 2. Children—Nutrition—Psychological aspects. 3. Eating disorders. I. Physicians Committee for Responsible Medicine.

RJ506.E18 H43 2001
613 .2'083—dc21   2001046860

Printed in the United States of America

10 9 8 7 6 5 4 3 2 1

Physicians Committee for
Responsible Medicine Expert Nutrition Panel

Healthy Eating for Life for Children

Neal D. Barnard, M.D.

Patricia Bertron, R.D.

Kathy Guillermo

Suzanne Havala, M.S., R.D., L.D.N., F.A.D.A.

Jennifer Keller, R.D.

Gabrielle Turner-McGrievy, M.S., R.D.

Vesanto Melina, M.S., R.D.

Kristine Kieswer

Martin Root, Ph.D.

with Amy Joy Lanou, Ph.D.

Contents

List of Recipes

Foreword

The writing of this book was motivated by the observation that many parents are unclear about how best to nourish their children at different stages of development. Well-intentioned parents like you want to do the very best for the long-term health and well-being of their children. They need help knowing where to begin.

Our hope is that by assembling an expert panel of doctors and nutritionists and by providing well-researched, easy-to-read information on healthy eating during childhood, we can help you promote excellent health for your children throughout their lives. Inside these pages you will find information organized into three sections: healthy eating guidelines for all the stages of childhood, nutrition-related topics of special concern to parents, and healthy recipes and menus for translating these principles into practice.

Chapters 1 and 2 offer a simple, new, healthier perspective on nutrition essentials. In chapters 3 through 8 you'll find a straightforward guide to healthy eating from conception to voting age. Nourishing your child is an once-in-a-lifetime opportunity. The foods you eat during pregnancy affect not only your child's development, but also health later in life. And the tastes your baby learns in early childhood will have a big influence on which foods he or she pulls from the refrigerator as a teenager or picks from a menu in adulthood. The food habits and attitudes your older children acquire will follow them into old age.

Children who learn to enjoy healthy foods have a tremendous asset. The nourishment you give your children now provides the raw materials they will use to grow. The right foods can help them stay slim and healthy, strengthen their immunity, reduce the risk of health problems later in life, and even boost their learning ability. It's easier than you might imagine. Healthy cooking and eating will soon be second nature for both you and your family.

Chapters 9 through 14 cover special topics in nutrition for children. In chapter 9 you'll learn about how food can affect common health problems. Unfortunately, many children get off on the wrong foot. If you could look into the arteries of children as young as three or four years, a surprising number have the early signs of artery changes that can lead to heart attacks later in life. Many children in Western countries have signs of heart disease by the time they reach their teens. Childhood also is the time when diet appears to have its greatest effect on later cancer risk, and often when weight problems begin. Diet can even alter the age at which puberty begins and can aggravate asthma, allergies, and other chronic childhood ailments.

Chapter 10 has the latest on how your child's eating habits affect learning ability. If you thought, for example, that sugar affects your child, you may be right. But there is much more to it, and we'll fill you in on what researchers know today about feeding the brain.

Young children in sports are different from adult athletes. Children not only need good nutrition to maximize performance but also need to continue to grow appropriately. If you are raising an athletic child, you'll want to pay special attention to chapter 11.

It is not easy to keep children on the right track. Parents face many challenges, from school lunch programs that do not always serve what you would like your children to have, to fast-food restaurants waiting for them on their way home, to endless television commercials pushing snacks and sodas. All these things affect our kids. All too often the result is overweight, a distorted body image, or even serious eating disorders. These are covered in chapters 12 to 14.

At the end you'll find a treasury of menus and delicious recipes based on the healthy guidelines outlined in this book. Developed by expert nutritionist, chef, and writer Jennifer Raymond, and later kid-tested and -approved, these tasty recipes will be sure to both please and nourish your child.

As you read this book and apply its concepts, keep in mind that many factors influence your child's food choices, from individual tastes to self-concept, beliefs about food, and health concerns. Then add to the mix the food attitudes learned from family and friends, the customs associated with specific events, and the need for food on the go—from vending machines and fast-food spots. The net result is that children sometimes make food choices we wish they hadn't. You can't possibly control all of these factors.

What you can do is prepare your children for navigating this minefield. That means offering them healthy choices early in life and helping them learn to make good decisions. Perhaps most importantly, you can set a good example with the healthy food choices you make yourself.

With the chance to enjoy healthy foods right from the start, your children will carry an important advantage throughout life. They are lucky to have you as a parent. Your desire to provide healthy meals will translate into a gift that lasts a lifetime.

A Note to the Reader

All children are individuals, and some have special medical needs. Neither this book nor any other takes the place of a pediatrician's advice.

At all stages of life, it is important to have complete nutrition. We recommend that all children, from toddlerhood on up, have a diet based on a variety of healthy vegetables, fruits, beans, and whole grains. It is essential to include a source of vitamin B_{12} (e.g., a children's multivitamin, B_{12}-fortified cereal, or B_{12}-fortified soy milk) as well as calcium-rich green leafy vegetables, beans, or, if you prefer, calcium-fortified fruit juices or soy milks.

Neal D. Barnard, M.D.
President, Physicians Committee
for Responsible Medicine

PART I

Essentials

1

Healthy Eating Basics

The world of nutrition has been revolutionized in recent years. While doctors and nutritionists used to promote eggs for protein, red meat for iron, and plenty of whole milk, they now sing the praises of leafy green vegetables, fresh fruit, beans, and whole grains. The fact is, the old way of eating has gotten us into trouble. Heart disease, cancer, and other problems have become epidemics, and our collective waistline is expanding, with no end in sight.

This is especially worrisome among kids. More and more children are struggling with their weight. Many have the high cholesterol levels doctors would expect to find in their out-of-shape parents. And when researchers look into these children's arteries, they find early signs of artery damage that are the first indications that the child will one day be headed for a heart attack.

Children are also growing up too fast. Puberty is occurring earlier and earlier. Not only does this open a Pandora's Box of psychological issues, it also increases cancer risk, as the hormones that are active during a woman's menstrual cycle are the same ones that fuel some cancers, including that of the breast.

Where are these changes coming from? The problem is not just that children are more sedentary than ever, fixed in place in front of TV screens and computers, driving instead of walking, and exercising less and less. The fact is, their diets are changing, and temptations are now everywhere. It is hard to turn on a children's television program without being assaulted by endless commercials for "fast foods" and snacks. And these foods are hard enough for some parents to resist, let alone their kids.

Hints of a healthier diet came from researchers who compared the eating habits in North America to those in China, Japan, Mediterranean countries, and Africa. Piecing together hundreds of studies, the pattern became clear. In countries where a healthy variety of whole grains, beans, vegetables, and fruits is consumed, children are much healthier than in those where children follow typical Western diets. Brag as we might about the meaty American diet, it is no match for the health power of the traditional foods of other lands. Japanese children, for example, have traditionally eaten rice, vegetables, and bean dishes, with much less meat than Westerners consume (and none at all in some religious traditions), virtually no dairy products, and very little oil. The payoff has come in the form of slim waistlines, enviably low cancer rates, and longevity that consistently outstrips that of Americans. A close look at kids with plentiful food in China, Thailand, Mexico, rural Africa, and elsewhere has helped nutrition authorities rewrite basic diet recommendations.

In 1998 Benjamin Spock, M.D., completely revised his book *Dr. Spock's Baby and Child Care,* the most influential parents' guide ever written and the biggest-selling book in history other than the Bible. Out with the fat and cholesterol and in with vegetables and fruits was his prescription. Never one to mince words, Dr. Spock recommended that parents raise children on a vegan diet—a diet made up entirely of plant foods with no meat (of any kind), eggs, or dairy products included. This event sparked a long-overdue review of current feeding practices for children. As the scientific studies and experiences of pediatricians were carefully evaluated, Dr. Spock was proven right: Vegetables, grains, legumes, and fruits are the optimal foods for both children and adults.

Why focus on these four food groups? Because they are cholesterol-free, high in fiber, low in fat, and rich in health-promoting substances found only in plants. They are also rich in healthy carbohydrates, proteins, vitamins, and minerals—the nutrients you and your family need. Foods from the plant kingdom are also excellent sources of protein and calcium—two nutrients once thought to be mainly in meat and dairy products.

In response to the new scientific understanding of the importance of the nutrients found in plants and the dangers of saturated fat and cholesterol, the Physicians Committee for Responsible Medicine developed the New Four Food Groups as a menu-planning guide in 1991. It is designed to be zero in cholesterol, low in fat, and fiber-rich to promote optimal health for you and your children. Since then it has proven to be an effective but very simple and practical guide for adults and children.

The serving numbers and sizes recommended for an average adult are shown on page 6. Throughout the upcoming pages, you will learn how to apply the New Four Food Groups to you and your children in different life stages including pregnancy, lactation, infancy, and all stages of childhood, from toddlerhood to the teen years.

This meal-planning guide is likely to introduce a few new tastes. But rest assured that with a little time, you will find eating from the New Four Food Groups easy, enjoyable, and wonderfully healthy.

Build your diet from these healthy foods. Keep in mind that the number of servings in each group is a minimum number. Add more servings as needed to meet your energy requirements. Small amounts of other foods such as nuts, seeds, oils, sweets, and processed foods can be part of a healthy diet; just be sure to focus your diet on the four food groups.

What do these food groups look like on your plate? When eating a pasta dish, choose a light marinara sauce instead of a meat or cream sauce. Or adorn your plate with vegetable lasagna, a bean burrito, baked beans, rice pilaf, or an autumn stew with mashed potatoes and plenty of vegetables. When it comes to soups, try lentil, split pea, minestrone, black bean, or vegetable soup. The recipe section in the last chapter will give you plenty of delicious ideas.

The New Four Food Groups

Vegetables: 3 or more servings a day

Serving size: 1 cup raw vegetables; ½ cup cooked vegetables

Vegetables provide vitamin C, beta-carotene, riboflavin, iron, calcium, fiber, and other nutrients. Dark green, leafy vegetables such as broccoli, collards, kale, mustard and turnip greens, chicory, and bok choy are especially good sources. Dark yellow and orange vegetables such as carrots, winter squash, sweet potatoes, and pumpkin provide extra beta-carotene.

Whole grains: 5 or more servings a day

Serving size: ½ cup hot cereal; 1 ounce dry cereal; 1 slice bread

This group includes bread, rice, pasta, hot or cold cereal, corn, millet, barley, bulgur, buckwheat groats, and tortillas. Whole grains are rich in fiber and other complex carbohydrates as well as protein, B vitamins, and zinc.

Fruit: 3 or more servings a day

Serving size: 1 medium piece fruit; ½ cup cooked fruit; 4 ounces juice

Fruits are rich in fiber, vitamin C, and beta-carotene. Be sure to include at least one serving each day of fruits that are high in vitamin C—citrus fruits, melons, and strawberries are all good choices. Choose whole fruit over fruit juices, which do not contain very much fiber.

Legumes: 2 or more servings a day

Serving size: ½ cup cooked beans; 4 ounces tofu or tempeh; 8 ounces soy milk

Legumes—another name for beans, peas, and lentils—are good sources of fiber, protein, iron, calcium, zinc, and B vitamins. This group also includes chickpeas, baked and refried beans, soy milk, tempeh, and textured vegetable protein.

Be sure to include a good source of vitamin B_{12} such as fortified cereals or vitamin supplements.

The Shift to Plant-Based Diets

Building your diet from grains, legumes, fruits, and vegetables, over the long run, has an enormous effect on your health and that of your loved ones. Here are a few of the advantages for your family.

Staying slim. A plant-based diet will help your children avoid the weight problems that will befall many of their classmates. That's a terrific advantage, because being overweight is a major contributor to diabetes, heart attack, stroke, cancer, and arthritis. Research studies show that vegetarians, on average, are 10 percent leaner than omnivores. Vegans are even leaner, weighing, on average, 12 to 20 pounds less than lacto-ovo vegetarians (i.e., vegetarians who eat eggs and dairy products) or omnivores.

A healthy heart. The foods you feed your children can keep their arteries open and healthy, nourishing their hearts and every other part of their bodies. Far too many children have the beginnings of serious heart disease before they finish high school.

Vegetarians have much lower cholesterol levels than nonvegetarians. Vegans (people who consume only foods from plant sources with no meat, fish, eggs, or dairy products) have even lower levels. These plant-based diets are dramatically better at reducing cholesterol levels than diets based on lean meats, chicken, or fish. The participants in Dr. Dean Ornish's history-making study at California's Preventive Medicine Research Institute lowered their cholesterol levels by a full 24 percent using a vegetarian diet and actually reversed their heart disease.

Protection from cancer. Though more common in adults, cancer can appear at any age. Raising your children on healthy meals will help protect them from this and other illnesses. Vegetarians are about 40 percent less likely to get cancer than nonvegetarians, regardless of other risks such as smoking, body size, and socioeconomic status. The vegetarians' advantage comes partly from what they're avoiding: One study found that eating just 1½ to 3 servings of meat, eggs, or dairy a week is associated with an increased incidence of breast cancer compared to eating less than 1 serving of these foods weekly.

Vegetarians also benefit from what they are including in their daily diets. Having generous amounts of fruits and vegetables every day helps protect against cancers in many sites, including the lung, breast, colon, bladder, stomach, and pancreas. Recent studies suggest that naturally occurring compounds in vegetables such as beta-carotene, lycopene, folic acid, and genistein, among many others, help ward off cancer. A study by Harvard University researchers of 109 breast biopsies showed that women whose breast tissue contained a high concentration of these helpful plant chemicals were 30 to 70 percent less likely to have breast cancer. In some cases natural antioxidants appear to help prevent and even repair the kinds of cell damage that can start the cancer process in the first place. Other plant nutrients, called phytoestrogens, which are particularly rich in soy products, can thereby reduce the cell-stimulating effects of sex hormones, in turn reducing the risk of hormone-related cancers such as breast, ovarian, or uterine cancer.

Healthy blood pressure. Building your kids' diet from the New Four Food Groups is great protection against high blood pressure, cutting the risk by nearly 70 percent. A study of African Americans found high blood pressure in 44 percent of nonvegetarians but in only 18 percent of vegetarians. Among a group of Caucasians, high blood pressure was found in 22 percent of meat-eaters compared to only 7 percent of vegetarians. The medical literature is full of studies showing that a vegetarian diet effectively and naturally lowers blood pressure.

Lower risk of diabetes. Diabetes is on the rise, especially in children. A person with diabetes has difficulty regulating blood sugar levels, and this can lead to a variety of problems, including impaired circulation, kidney disease, strokes, and heart attacks. Vegetarians are much less likely to develop diabetes, and this same diet has even been shown to be effective in treating, and sometimes reversing Type 2 (adult-onset) diabetes.

In addition to keeping you slim and free of these major chronic diseases, building your diet from the New Four Food Groups has other advantages for children and adults. Vegetarians have been shown in several studies to gain a measure of protection from kidney stones and other kidney diseases, gallstones, diverticulosis, appendicitis, constipation, and hemorrhoids, among other conditions. There is no longer any question: The healthiest diets are built from the New Four Food Groups. When your children are in the habit of eating healthy foods, they are on track for long, healthy lives.

2

Nutrients and Where to Find Them

W ith any diet change comes the question "Will my family get all the nutrition we need?" Here's a quick run-down on nutrients and where you'll find them.

Protein

Protein is used for growth and repair in the body. The best way to ensure adequate protein in the diet is to eat daily servings of whole grains such as cereals, brown rice, and whole wheat bread; legumes such as peas and black beans; and a variety of vegetables and fruits. Soy products such as tofu and soy milk are also rich sources of protein, although they are by no means the only ones. Of course, all of these foods provide much more than just protein; they also contain fiber, vitamins, and minerals, and healthful complex carbohydrates.

The American Dietetic Association and the U.S. government both hold, in their official nutrition policies, that a varied diet of foods from plants has plenty of protein. While some have advocated "combining" or "complementing" proteins, for example, by eating grains and legumes at the same meal, we now recognize that this occurs naturally with a varied diet drawn from plant foods, and there is no need to carefully combine foods for protein.

Meats and eggs are very high in protein, but this is hardly an advantage. In fact, we're now seeing how dangerous this can be. Most meat-eaters actually get more than twice the protein their bodies need, overworking their kidneys and increasing their risk of serious kidney disease. High-protein foods also encourage the loss of calcium, which passes from the bones into the bloodstream, then through the kidneys into the urine. This is due not only to the amount of protein in animal products but also to the type of protein they contain. Meat, eggs, and dairy proteins are rich in sulfur-containing amino acids, which are especially likely to carry calcium out through the kidneys. The end result is that people on high-protein diets— not simply the ultra-high-protein diets marketed for weight loss, but even the typical American diet—are more likely to get kidney stones and to suffer from osteoporosis as they get older. Large research studies show that populations with the greatest protein intake have the most bone breaks later in life.

Complex Carbohydrates

Complex carbohydrates, or starches, provide the energy that keeps you going. Not surprisingly, active children need more of this important nutrient than adult family members who sit in front of a TV or a computer for hours on end. Found in vegetables, fruits, grains, and beans, carbohydrates are burned by the body as fuel, much as a car burns gasoline. The term "complex carbohydrate" means that the starch molecule consists of many sugars wound together. They are released gradually during digestion to supply energy over a few hours' time. In contrast, sugar, honey, corn syrup, and other common sweeteners are simple carbohydrates that provide fuel in a form that is quickly absorbed and does not last. These sweets also contain no fiber, vitamins, minerals, or other substances that benefit the body.

Fats and Essential Fatty Acids

In large doses, fat is truly our enemy, not only where our figures are concerned, but also for our hearts and other organs. In small amounts it can be our friend, and, in fact, is essential. The essential fats come in two types:

1. Omega-3 oils are found in many vegetables, fruits, and beans and in a more concentrated form in flaxseed oil, soybean products (e.g., tofu), corn oil, canola oil, and wheat germ oil.
2. Omega-6 oils are found in many plant foods and in a concentrated form in borage, evening primrose, black currant, and hemp oils.

The omega-3 and omega-6 fatty acids are important for growth and proper development and are involved in the normal functioning of all tissues of the body. If intake of these essential fatty acids is too low in the diet, the result can be reduced growth rate, decreased immune function, abnormalities in the liver and kidney, and dry and scaly skin. A diet rich in fruits, vegetables, and legumes will help your family members get the essential fatty acids needed. A simple way to give your diet an omega-3 boost is to add a small amount of flaxseed oil to your salad dressing or to sprinkle some ground flaxseeds in your morning cereal or fruit smoothie.

Fiber

Fiber is the roughage in fruits, grains, vegetables, and legumes that resists digestion. Fiber has many important functions, and researchers are learning more and more about the value of this powerful part of plant-based foods. For example, the soluble fiber in oats and beans reduces cholesterol levels, so it is a useful factor in the prevention of heart disease. Insoluble fiber, found in wheat and other cereal grains, helps keep the digestive tract working well, prevents constipation, and reduces the risk of colon cancer. Fiber also helps the body eliminate wastes and toxins that are filtered from the bloodstream by the liver and secreted into the intestinal tract. Foods without fiber, such as meat, dairy products, eggs, and refined grains, stay in the lower intestine longer, slow down digestion, and work against these important waste-removal processes.

Calcium

In addition to being an important building block of bones and teeth, calcium has a host of other important uses in the body. It helps maintain blood pressure and is involved in muscle contraction, nerve transmission, and blood clotting. As noted above, the amount of calcium retained by the body is influenced by protein. Eliminating animal protein typically cuts calcium losses in half, so when animal proteins are replaced with plant proteins, the body actually needs less calcium.

Even so, we do need calcium in our daily diets. Leafy green vegetables such as broccoli, kale, collards, and bok choy are rich in calcium. The exception is spinach, which contains a large amount of calcium but holds on to it very tenaciously, so less of it is absorbed into the body.

Beans also supply plenty of calcium. There are more than 100 milligrams of calcium in a plate of vegetarian baked beans. Chickpeas, pinto and white beans, tofu, and other beans and bean products are good sources, too. These foods also contain magnesium, which your body uses along with calcium to build bones.

Fortified foods are another useful source. Calcium-fortified orange and apple juices are rich in highly absorbable calcium—300 milligrams or even more calcium per cup. Soy milk, rice milk, and other nondairy milks made from oats or even almonds are also widely available; check the label to find a calcium-rich brand. More and more breakfast cereals are becoming significant sources of calcium as well.

CALCIUM IN FOODS (IN MILLIGRAMS)

FOOD (SERVING SIZE)	CALCIUM
Apricots (3 medium raw)	15
Black turtle beans (1 cup, boiled)	102
Broccoli (1 cup, chopped, frozen, boiled)	94
Brown rice (1 cup, long-grain, cooked)	20
Brussels sprouts (1 cup, fresh, boiled)	56
Butternut squash (1 cup, cubes, baked)	84
Chickpeas (1 cup, boiled)	80
Collards (1 cup, chopped, frozen, boiled)	358
Dates (10 medium dried)	27

English muffin (plain)	99
Figs (10 medium dried)	269
Great Northern beans (1 cup, boiled)	120
Green beans (1 cup, boiled)	58
Kale (1 cup boiled)	94
Lentils (1 cup, boiled)	38
Lima beans (1 cup, boiled)	32
Mustard greens (1 cup, chopped, frozen, boiled)	152
Navel orange (1 medium)	52
Navy beans (1 cup, boiled)	127
Oatmeal (2 packets, instant)	326
Orange juice, calcium-fortified (8 oz)	300
Peas (1 cup, frozen, boiled)	38
Pinto beans (1 cup, boiled)	82
Raisins (⅔ cup)	53
Soybeans (1 cup, boiled)	175
Spinach (1 cup, boiled)	244
Sweet potato (1 cup, mashed, boiled)	68
Swiss chard (1 cup, boiled)	102
Tofu, calcium-set (½ cup, raw, firm)	258
Vegetarian baked beans (1 cup)	127
White beans (1 cup, boiled)	161

Source: J. A. T. Pennington, *Bowes and Church's Food Values of Portions Commonly Used,* 17th ed. (Philadelphia: J. B. Lippincott, 1998).

Iron

Iron is essential to our red blood cells, carrying into our cells the life-giving oxygen from the air we breathe. Iron deficiency can cause lethargy, apathy, inability to concentrate, a tendency to feel cold, and loss of productivity. Maintaining adequate iron stores is important, especially for pregnant women and small children post-weaning. But don't go overboard. Too much can be toxic.

How do you find the perfect balance? Most days simply eat lots of vegetables and beans. Broccoli, collards, squash, and soy, navy, and Great Northern beans are great sources. Add some vitamin C–rich foods and you will increase iron absorption further. Broccoli, rich in both vitamin C and iron, does double duty in this case. So move the steamed broccoli from the side of your family's plate up to front and center. You and your children can even get your iron from your morning bowl of cereal, as many are now fortified with iron.

While there is iron in meats, along with plenty of fat and cholesterol, iron's structure is such that it overloads your system with higher and higher doses, no matter how much you already have. The result is that meats can contribute to iron overload. Plant iron, on the other hand, contributes what your body needs without the dangerous excesses. With children, the tables are turned. Dairy products reduce their iron absorption by irritating the digestive tract and causing the gradual loss of iron-rich red blood cells.

Studies show that populations that consume few or no animal products actually have equal or greater iron intake than meat-eaters, so vegan children who are fed healthy diets are not at risk of iron deficiency.

Zinc

Zinc works with proteins to foster proper growth and development. It is found in rice, corn, oats, various other grains, spinach, mushrooms, potatoes, peas, and beans, as well as whole-grain breads and breakfast cereals. Studies have shown that vegetarian and omnivorous diets provide similar amounts of zinc. As with iron, consuming too much zinc, especially from supplements, is potentially dangerous. If you use zinc lozenges when you feel a cold coming on, limit your use to three or fewer days.

Vitamins

Children require vitamins in small amounts to grow and stay healthy. Most are readily found in foods, although there is an important role for supplements of vitamins B_{12} and sometimes D, as you can see in the following table.

VITAMIN GUIDE

VITAMIN	WHAT IT DOES	HOW TO GET IT
Vitamin A and beta-carotene, its precursor	<ul><li>important for good vision</li><li>ensures the health of intestinal and bronchial linings, as well as the urinary system and skin</li><li>aids bone and tooth growth</li><li>necessary for the immune system, the body's defense against infection</li><li>important for growth and reproduction</li><li>protects against cancer</li></ul>	Vitamin A's precursor, beta-carotene, is found in yellow and orange vegetables, such as carrots, pumpkins, squash, and sweet potatoes, as well as in green vegetables. Beta-carotene is naturally converted into vitamin A by the body.
Thiamin, also called vitamin B_1	<ul><li>important for metabolism—using energy from foods</li><li>supports the nervous system</li><li>supports normal appetite</li></ul>	Thiamin is widespread in whole plant foods. Whole grains, vegetables, and beans are good sources. Polished rice, white flour, and other processed grains lose thiamin, but many commercially prepared foods are enriched with thiamin.
Riboflavin, also called vitamin B_2	<ul><li>important for metabolism—using energy from foods</li><li>supports normal vision and skin health</li></ul>	Riboflavin is found in leafy green vegetables, whole grains, and enriched breads and cereals.

VITAMIN	WHAT IT DOES	HOW TO GET IT
Niacin, also called vitamin B_3	• important for metabolism—using energy from foods • supports health of the skin and the nervous and digestive systems	Whole grains, enriched breads and cereals, nuts, and beans are good sources of niacin.
Vitamin B_6, also called pyridoxine	• important for metabolism—using energy from fat and protein • helps to make red blood cells	Vitamin B_6 is plentiful in corn, oats, cabbage, bananas, green and leafy vegetables, cantaloupes, split peas and other legumes, and wheat bran.
Folic acid, also called folate	• required to make all new cells, especially red blood cells • helps the body to replicate and repair DNA • very important to growing fetuses, as well as to growing toddlers	Folic acid–rich foods include strawberries, cantaloupes, whole grains, spinach, broccoli, turnip greens, other leafy green vegetables, legumes, and seeds.
Vitamin B_{12}, also called cobalamin	• used in new cell synthesis • essential for healthy nerves and blood	Cereals or nondairy milks that have been enriched with B_{12} or nutritional yeast are good sources. All common multivitamins contain B_{12} and

Vitamin	What It Does	How to Get It
Vitamin B$_{12}$ *(continued)*		provide the most reliable and convenient source. Vitamin B$_{12}$ is made by bacteria. Animal products contain B$_{12}$ made by bacteria in the animal's gut, but are not preferred sources due to their fat and cholesterol.
Vitamin D	• necessary for the body's proper utilization of calcium in bone	The body manufactures vitamin D when the skin is exposed to sunshine. Twenty minutes of sunshine on the arms and face every day is usually enough. Children and adults who have dark skin may need more sunshine, as the pigment in their skin is effective at blocking the sun's rays. Supplements or supplemented foods such as soy milk or cereal may be needed in very cold or cloudy climates where sun exposure is limited.

VITAMIN	WHAT IT DOES	HOW TO GET IT
Vitamin E	• helps maintain healthy skin • protects cells and membranes • helps defend the body against disease • needed for normal nerve development	Vitamin E is found in many foods, including whole grains, spinach, broccoli, and other leafy green vegetables, corn, cucumbers, nuts, seeds, and vegetable oils. Highly processed foods and fried foods lose their vitamin E during processing.
Vitamin K	• important for blood clotting • helps regulate blood calcium levels	Vitamin K is found in dark, leafy green vegetables and is made by intestinal bacteria. Infants are often given a one-time supplement at birth.

Source: E. M. N. Hamilton, E. N. Whitney, and F. S. Sizer. *Nutrition Concepts and Controversies,* 6th ed. (St. Paul, Minn.: West, 1994).

Vitamins are crucial for children in all stages of growth and development. Still, it is possible to have too much of a good thing. A supplement that has no more than 100 percent of the recommended dietary allowance for each included vitamin is generally okay. But babies, toddlers, and children should not be given large doses of vitamin supplements, as they can be toxic and cause serious illness. Vitamins A, D, and K can be particularly dangerous if they are given improperly. Always ask your pediatrician or a dietitian about supplements you may be considering.

What about Meat, Dairy, and Eggs?

While it is true that meat contains protein, that is just part of the story. All meats, including poultry and fish, contain significant amounts of cholesterol and saturated fat. Dairy products and eggs are problematic for many of the same reasons. Even the leanest cuts of meat are surprisingly high in saturated fat, increasing the risk of artery blockages, which start in childhood and easily lead to heart disease later in life.

Cholesterol is found only in animal products, so abstaining from meat, dairy, and eggs completely eliminates cholesterol from the diet. Our bodies make all the cholesterol we need, so avoiding dietary sources can only benefit us. As mentioned above, studies comparing people who eat meat with those who eat vegetarian foods show that vegetarians have decidedly lower levels of cholesterol and a much lower risk of heart disease.

Even small portions of meat eaten regularly can be damaging to the heart. Dr. Dean Ornish, renowned for his work with heart disease patients, demonstrated that a low-fat vegetarian diet, exercise, and stress reduction can actually reverse decades' worth of plaque built up in the arteries. And the only "side effects" his patients experienced were weight loss, more energy, and a new lease on life.

Time and again, when researchers look at diets around the world, they see countries with the highest meat and dairy consumption suffering from cancer, heart disease, diabetes, and obesity. Even in China, where everyone eats less meat than in North America, the Chinese eating a bit more meat get more diseases.

Imagine the effect that a lifetime of healthy, vegan eating would have on the next generation. Children would be slimmer, healthier, and much less likely to be threatened with heart disease, cancer, food allergies, diabetes, or obesity. A vegan diet is the most powerful protection against chronic disease we can offer our children.

Hidden Dangers in Meats

Aside from fat and cholesterol, meats also contain cancer-causing chemicals, like those in cigarette smoke, that form as proteins are cooked. These carcinogens, called heterocyclic amines, are found in all cooked meats, including fish, white and red meats, and poultry. The amount in grilled chicken, in fact, is fifteen times higher than in hamburger or steak.

Cow's Milk: No Longer Recommended

Perhaps the most surprising—and still controversial—area in the science of nutrition concerns dairy products. Needless to say, whole milk, cheese, sour cream, and ice cream are high in cholesterol and saturated fat. But concerns also have emerged not just about the *amount* of fat in dairy, but also about the *type*. Dairy products simply do not contain the proper combination of fats for human development. This is why manufacturers replace milk fat with vegetable oils in preparing infant formulas. But even for children beyond infancy, dairy products still contain the wrong type of fats needed for healthy development. As we've seen, you'll find small amounts of essential fat in foods such as beans, grains, flax seeds, avocados, nut butters, tofu, and other soy products.

Cow's milk contains proteins that may cause or aggravate a variety of conditions, from asthma to canker sores, constipation to recurrent ear infections. More seriously, milk can contribute to iron deficiency and anemia. Perhaps most worrisome of all, more than ninety studies have investigated the link between insulin-dependent (Type 1) diabetes and proteins in dairy products. We now understand that giving cow's milk to babies and children can cause their immune systems to react to its proteins, forming antibodies against them, which later destroy their own insulin-producing cells—the start of lifelong Type 1 diabetes. To avoid this, simply wean your child from breast milk to soy formula or soy milk and pass up using cow's milk altogether. More information on the benefits of nondairy milks can be found in chapter 5.

The Problem with Fish

The negative sides of other meats, eggs, and dairy emerged slowly in recent decades, but fish is still trying to slip through with a squeaky-clean image. But ask a pediatric researcher about eating fish, and a whole new picture emerges. You may have heard that pregnant women are urged to avoid fish (see chapter 3 for more details) due to its frequent contamination with chemicals in the environment. The same goes for your child after he or she is born. Contamination has become a serious problem, primarily because inland waterways and oceans have become civilization's sewers.

Chemicals from factories, pesticide runoff from farm fields, city sewage, livestock manure, and many other pollutants drain into streams and rivers and are carried to the oceans. Fish absorb these contaminants as water passes through their gills. Larger fish take in even more chemicals when they eat smaller fish.

Tests conducted by *Consumer Reports* found PCBs—industrial chemicals used in electrical equipment—in 25 percent of swordfish, 43 percent of salmon, and 50 percent of whitefish. PCBs accumulate in a fish's body and also accumulate in the body of the person who eats that fish. And they stay there. This is bad news, because PCBs are linked to cancer, and, like most carcinogens, are especially dangerous to growing children.

Like PCBs, mercury from factories settles in waterways. Ninety percent of swordfish are contaminated with this deadly element, according to the *Consumer Reports* study, and a typical can of tuna sitting on a grocery store shelf contains about 15 micrograms of mercury. The FDA issued a warning to parents stating that pregnant and breastfeeding mothers as well as small children should avoid eating shark, swordfish, king mackerel, and tilefish due to the high levels of mercury found in these large fish.

There is no need for anyone to risk mercury poisoning; the essential fatty acids found in fish are available in vegetable oils and also can be consumed in pill form.

The Safety of Vegan Diets

With all the information now available about the long-term health benefits of diets built from vegetables, grains, legumes, and fruits, there really is no question about whether a vegan diet is safe. The American Dietetic Association's official position paper on vegetarian diets clearly states, "Appropriately planned vegan and lacto-ovo-vegetarian [vegetarians who consume dairy and eggs] diets satisfy nutrient needs of infants, children, and adolescents and promote normal growth." Vegan diets are not only nutritionally adequate, they also offer significant nutritional advantages to growing bodies. And, as you will see in chapter 10, vegan diets may be the best food for developing minds as well. One study showed that veg-

Nutritional Advantages of the New Four Food Groups

- cholesterol-free
- low in saturated fat and total fat
- high in fiber
- high in the antioxidants: vitamin C, vitamin E, and beta-carotene
- high in the B vitamins: folate, thiamin, and riboflavin
- high in protective substances called phytochemicals
- adequate in protein, iron, and calcium, and free from animal protein

etarian children had a mean IQ well above average, and mental age advanced a year ahead of chronological age, providing reassurance that vegetarian diets provide for normal brain development.

Still, it is important to plan for complete nutrition, especially for vitamin B_{12}. A wholesome variety of foods from the New Four Food Groups, plus a daily vitamin or one or more servings of a fortified food, provide a balanced and very healthy diet.

Getting Started

Once you start experimenting with healthy foods, you will find food preparation easy and your meals satisfying. And many people experience pleasant surprises when they shift to a healthy, vegan diet. Some find that they lose those twenty pounds they have been trying to shed for the past few years; others find their allergies begin to ease; some find that their skin is clearer or that they have more energy. Whatever your personal experience is, you will get the added satisfaction of knowing that you are offering your children optimal nutrition and a chance to develop the tastes that will protect them throughout their lives.

PART II

Making It Work for You

3

Starting Life Well: Nutrition in Pregnancy

A Healthy Pregnancy—A Good Place to Start

Thinking about having a baby? If so, now is the perfect time to take a fresh look at your lifestyle habits and consider whether they are providing what you need for a healthy pregnancy. What's good for your developing baby, before birth and after, is good for you as well. Beginning a pregnancy with a fit body and a healthy eating style will give you and your child a head start to lifelong good health. In fact, the foods you eat during pregnancy as well as those you give your child in the first year of life have an impact on health—not just during the developmental years but also into his or her forties, fifties, and beyond.

Your fitness level is important, too. Women who start their pregnancy at a healthy body weight and body composition are better prepared for the physical challenge of making another person and are less at risk for complications such as hypertension, diabetes, miscarriage, stillbirth, and others. Regular exercisers who continue their physical activity with care during their pregnancies have been shown to have healthier pregnancies than less active women.

Exercise in Pregnancy

Doctors used to recommend that women discontinue vigorous activity while pregnant. But today we know that women who continue their exercise programs (sometimes slightly modified versions) benefit greatly, provided there are no contraindications. Exercise offers mothers improved cardiovascular function, limited weight gain, easier and less complicated labor, quick recovery, and improved fitness, not to mention a better state of mind. Exercise during pregnancy has some benefits for your baby, too. These may include improved stress tolerance and leaner bodies as toddlers. Even sedentary women would do well to walk or begin other low-intensity activities to attain some of these benefits, provided their pregnancies are free of complications.

Talk to your doctor or an exercise specialist to plan an exercise program appropriate for your needs. Look for an exercise trainer who has been certified by the American College of Sports Medicine (www.ascm.org). You'll feel better for it!

Also important throughout life, but especially important during pregnancy and breastfeeding, is avoiding toxic substances such as alcohol, tobacco, certain drugs, pesticides, and hormones and environmental toxins found in meat and fish, as we'll see later in this chapter.

If all this sounds like a tall order—eating right, exercising, staying vigilant about alcohol, while you're also managing all the other challenges pregnancy brings—take heart. You can do it. And the payoff is enormous, for both you and your baby. Some of these good habits might even rub off on the rest of the family, too.

Luckily, eating well during pregnancy is not all that different from eating well throughout life. It's just more important, because you are not only providing yourself the nutrients needed for health and energy, you are also providing your child with all the building blocks and energy he or she needs to become a healthy newborn. Meals based on a variety of whole grains, legumes, fruits, and vegetables are your best choice. Add small quantities of nuts and seeds and a source of vitamin B_{12} from fortified cereal, fortified soy milk, or a vitamin supplement, and you and your developing baby will have all the nutrients needed.

During your pregnancy you will need to eat a little more food than usual and pay a little added attention to consuming nutrient-rich foods. Requirements for some nutrients such as folate, iron, calcium, and vitamin B_{12} are higher while you are pregnant because they are essential for proper fetal development.

Eating for Two

On average, pregnant women are encouraged to gain only two to four pounds for the first trimester of pregnancy. Thereafter a healthy weight gain will be roughly 1 to $1\frac{1}{2}$ pounds per week. Of course, there is always some variation among women and from week to week. This means that some weeks you might not gain anything and other weeks you may gain 2 or 3 pounds.

In 1990, the Institute of Medicine of the National Academy of Sciences set guidelines for weight gain during pregnancy. These recommendations, to gain between 15 and 45 pounds, are based on your prepregnancy weight. Shorter women (5'2" and under) should plan for gains at the low end of these ranges. In a recent report, scientists confirmed that these recommended gains are associated with the best outcomes for both mother and child. Unfortunately, only 30 to 40 percent of women in the populations studied achieved pregnancy weight gain that fell within these ranges—the rest gained either too little or too much.

The take-home message regarding weight gain during pregnancy is to strive for a weight gain that falls within the ranges shown in table on page 28. This will help reduce your risk of premature birth, poor fetal growth, the need for cesarean birth, and postpartum weight retention.

During pregnancy you are "eating for two," but keep in mind that one of you is very small during this entire period—only growing to be 6 to 10 pounds by the end of nine months. This means that while your energy needs are increasing during pregnancy, it is only by a small amount. During the first month of pregnancy, no additional calories are needed. In the remaining eight months, a pregnant woman needs, on average, about 250 to 300 additional calories every day.

When it comes to calories, quality, not quantity, is what matters

Recommended Total Weight Gain during Pregnancy

CURRENT WEIGHT GAIN RECOMMENDATIONS

Normal-weight women	25 to 35 lbs
Underweight women (<90% of desirable weight)	28 to 40 lbs
Overweight women (>120% of desirable weight)	15 to 25 lbs
Obese women (>135% of desirable weight)	15 lbs
Adolescent women	30 to 45 lbs
Normal-weight women carrying twins	35 to 45 lbs

most. It's best to choose these extra calories from healthy plant sources. Try a vibrant salad of spinach leaves, fresh tomatoes, and oranges. Keep fruits such as apples, bananas, and pears with you when you are on the go. Center your meals on wholesome brown rice, noodles, or protein-rich legumes. You can get the extra 250 to 300 calories you'll need each day from as little as a cup of baked beans, a cup and a half of brown rice, or three servings of fruits and vegetables. These healthy low-fat foods also provide the extra protein, minerals, and vitamins a future mom needs and require little or no planning. Try to avoid "junk" foods such as a candy bar or a soda, which would provide calories without the nutrients.

Meal Planning

When planning your daily menu during pregnancy, the most important thing to keep in mind is that meals built from grains, legumes, vegetables, and fruits are an effective and delicious choice for meeting your nutrient needs. Many doctors feel, for the reasons discussed in chapter 1, that choosing a diet of plant-based foods is the healthiest, and often simplest, way to provide everything your growing baby needs and to maximize your health in the process.

Because pregnant women have higher requirements for some nutrients, some care in choosing your daily menu is recommended.

To make this easier, a group of registered dietitians with the American Dietetic Association put together daily meal planning guidelines for pregnant women. These guidelines may be a little different from what you are used to, but rest assured that a menu made up of whole foods, largely or entirely from plant sources, is an excellent way to give your body, and that of your developing child, the good nutrition needed.

DAILY MEAL PLANNING GUIDELINES FOR PREGNANT WOMEN

Whole grains, breads, cereals: 7 or more servings Choose whole grains whenever possible.	Serving: 1 slice bread, ½ bun or bagel, ½ cup cooked cereal, grain, or pasta, ¾ to 1 cup ready-to-eat cereal
Legumes, nuts, seeds, nondairy milks: 5 or more servings Choose calcium-rich foods such as fortified soy milk, tofu, and beans often.	Serving: ½ cup cooked beans, 4 oz tempeh or tofu, 3 oz meat analogue, 2 tbsp nuts, seeds, nut or seed butter, 1 cup fortified soy milk or other nondairy milk
Vegetables: 4 or more servings Choose at least one dark green vegetable daily. Broccoli, kale, collard greens, mustard greens, and bok choy are good calcium-rich vegetables and should be selected often.	Serving: ½ cup cooked or 1 cup raw
Fruits: 4 or more servings Chooose fresh fruit and calcium-fortified juices often.	Serving: ½ cup canned fruit or juice or 1 medium fruit, or 1 cup fruit pieces

Source: Adapted from a Vegetarian Nutrition Dietetic Practice Group, American Dietetic Association, 1996.

Meeting Nutrient Needs

In this section we'll look at the special nutrient needs you'll have during pregnancy. Luckily, it turns out that if you follow the straightforward meal planning guidelines described here and include a serving of a vitamin B_{12}-fortified food or take a vitamin B_{12} supplement, you do not have to concern yourself with each individual nutrient.

Protein

Protein is used to make new cells, so it makes sense that your need for protein increases when you are providing nutrients for a growing fetus. You will need about 10 grams a day more protein than you normally do. It is easy to meet this requirement, with as little as a cup of peas, a small bowl of black bean soup or chili, a bagel, or a handful of mixed nuts. In fact, most women who consume enough calories already consume more than enough protein—whether they follow a healthy plant-based diet or a mixed diet. This is because we only need a small amount of our energy as protein (10 to 15% of calories), and most of the whole foods we eat—even vegetables— contain at least this amount. Many plant-based foods are protein-rich and have more than 10 percent of calories from protein.

A few foods have very little protein, such as fruit (bananas 4%, peaches 6%) and fruit juices (apple juice 1%, orange juice 6%). Others have almost no protein at all, such as most candy, soda, salad dressings, condiments such as jelly and catsup, spices, oils, and margarine. Meat and dairy products have a lot of protein (ranging from 20 to 50% of calories as protein) but contain high amounts of fat and cholesterol as well, which are not healthy for adults or a growing fetus. Oftentimes, diets that contain meat and dairy are too high in protein, which can be harmful as well. For example, meat-rich diets cause you to excrete more calcium in the urine, thus upsetting your body's calcium balance. So, to meet your increased protein needs during pregnancy, you simply need to choose a variety of whole plant foods, eat enough food to meet your energy demands, and avoid consuming large quantities of the zero-protein foods.

PERCENTAGE OF CALORIES AS PROTEIN IN PLANT FOODS

PROTEIN-RICH PLANT FOODS	PROTEIN (% OF CALORIES)
Spinach	49
Broccoli	48
Asparagus	44
Tofu	43
Mushrooms	38
Green beans	25
Canned beans	21
Bean soup	20
Tomatoes	19
Sesame seeds	18
Vegetable juice	18
Peanut butter	18
Oatmeal	17
Mixed grain bread	15
Noodles	14
Raisin bran cereal	14
Fresh corn	13
Beets	13
Vegetable soup	12
Almonds	12
Corn tortillas	12
Baked squash	11
Baked potato	11
Carrots	10

Fewer Pregnancy Complications for Vegetarian Moms?

In a 1987 study of seventeen hundred pregnancies at a vegan community in Tennessee in the southeastern United States, problems during pregnancy were extremely rare. In twenty years there was only one case of preeclampsia, a condition involving hypertension, fluid retention, urinary protein loss, and excessive weight gain. By contrast, preeclampsia occurs in at least 2 percent of all pregnancies in the United States. And only one in a hundred babies had to be delivered by cesarean section, compared with much higher rates in the general population. Other researchers have reported similar results.

Essential Fatty Acids

The human body has a very low requirement for fat, because we can make most types of fat from the excess energy in the food we eat. There are, however, a few types of fats that we need for growth and health that we have to get from the food we eat—these are the essential fatty acids (EFAs). Recent research suggests that pregnant women may have increased needs for these fatty acids, as they are needed for fetal growth, brain development, learning, and behavior.

Two key essential fatty acids (linoleic acid and α-linolenic acid) are mostly found in seeds and seed oils and in the green leaves of plants. These two EFAs can be converted into other important fatty acids, albeit rather slowly. They are also present in fatty fish, but this is not a recommended source of EFAs for pregnant women because fish often contain high levels of environmental contaminants along with saturated fat and cholesterol.

To offer your growing fetus an adequate supply of these EFAs without consuming too much fat or toxins, some doctors recommend a supplement containing a mixture of essential fatty acids. An alternative is to make salad dressing with flaxseed oil or to incorporate it into your menus by sprinkling the seeds on your morning cereal or by blending them in a frozen fruit smoothie for an afternoon snack. In addition, you should limit your intake of margarine and other foods containing highly processed fats, as the trans-fatty acids in these foods have been shown to reduce EFAs.

Mighty Minerals: Calcium, Iron, and Zinc

Minerals are the building blocks of many body systems. Three in particular—calcium, iron, and zinc—merit special attention during pregnancy, as they play a crucial role in healthy fetal development.

Calcium is needed to build bones and teeth, so your growing fetus will benefit from your attention to eating calcium-rich foods. With just four or more servings of foods such as calcium-processed tofu, kale, collards, bok choy, broccoli, beans, figs, sunflower seeds, tahini, almond butter, and calcium-fortified soy milk, juices, and cereals, you will easily meet your requirement. The hormonal changes in your body during pregnancy help you to absorb calcium more effectively and ensure that your growing baby gets enough of this important nutrient. If your diet is very low in calcium, it's your bones rather than your baby's that will suffer. If you are under twenty-five years of age and have trouble consuming enough calcium-rich foods or are at risk for osteoporosis, a calcium supplement of 400 to 600 mg a day may be recommended by your doctor. If so, be sure to take your calcium supplement with meals and at a different time than any other supplements you might take.

Milk and other dairy products were once thought to be the ideal sources of calcium. But extensive research accumulated in the past twenty-five years has revealed how wrong we were. Milk and other dairy products are rich in animal protein, which causes your body to excrete more calcium than you would if you were eating plant foods. So when you drink milk, you are taking in calcium, but also losing it at the same time. Also, many adults have difficulty digesting milk—either because they've lost the enzyme lactase needed to break down milk sugar, or because they are allergic to one or more substances in milk. In fact, most of the world's population cannot digest milk after infancy. "Lactose intolerance," as it has come to be known, causes intestinal distress, including diarrhea, constipation, gas, bloating, and stomach pain. In light of this, many doctors now recommend plant sources of calcium to meet calcium needs during pregnancy. (See the table "Calcium in Foods" in chapter 2 for good sources.)

Your need for iron is high during pregnancy because your body makes more blood to take nutrients and oxygen to the fetus, and you need iron available to make fetal blood. Consumption of iron-rich foods such as whole grains, legumes, tofu, leafy green vegetables, and fortified breakfast cereals is important throughout pregnancy and especially during the last trimester, when iron needs are highest. You'll absorb more iron from these foods if you have a vitamin C–rich food such as orange juice, tomatoes, or peppers at the same meal. A black bean burrito with tomato salsa or cereal and orange juice are great combinations.

Some women may not have adequate stores of iron, particularly during the second half of pregnancy, and may need a supplement of 30 milligrams a day. Women who are large, anemic, or pregnant with twins may need a 60-milligram supplement. However, most women, especially those who eat a variety of vegetables, fruits, legumes, and grains, have enough iron stored in their bodies and do not need supplementation. Indeed, some recent studies show that too much iron may increase the risk of complications and may prolong pregnancy. Some researchers now believe that the level of iron recommended during pregnancy is too high. The best way to find out whether you need to take an iron supplement is to have a simple iron blood test, called a ferritin test, at the beginning and middle of pregnancy. An iron supplement can then be prescribed if needed.

Zinc is essential for growth and development. Ideally you'll want to consume 50 percent more of it throughout your pregnancy. Even a mild zinc deficiency, which is common among women, has been linked to complications in labor and delivery. Legumes, nuts, whole grains, and cereals are good sources of zinc. If you want to increase the amount of zinc you absorb from these foods, try bean sprouts, sprouted grains, or yeast-raised breads.

When considering these important minerals, keep in mind that when you choose a plant-based diet, including a variety of foods from all of the New Four Food Groups—vegetables, fruits, legumes, and grains—you will meet all your mineral needs with ease. By building your daily menu around whole foods that include lots of vegetables and legumes while you are pregnant, you will not have to plan for each of these nutrients individually.

Vitamin Watch: Folate, Vitamin B$_{12}$, and Vitamin D

Vitamins, in minuscule quantities, are vital to life. Three vitamins warrant special mention: folate, vitamin D, and vitamin B$_{12}$. By choosing a plant-based diet and supplementing it with fortified cereals, fortified soy milk, or a multivitamin, it's quite easy to meet your needs for these vitamins as well as all the other nutrients you need to grow a healthy baby.

Folate, also called folic acid, is necessary for the development of the your baby's nervous system, among other functions. In fact, it is especially important in the first three to four weeks of pregnancy, when the neural tube is developing. This tube of nerves later becomes the spinal cord. Without adequate folate present at this time, the neural tube may not close properly and can result in neural tube defects. Many people, especially those who eat meat, dairy, eggs, and processed foods daily, do not consume enough folate in their diets. Folate gets its name from the word "foliage" because it is found in the leaves of many plants. Dark green, leafy vegetables and legumes are especially rich, so women who eat meals containing lots of these foods have no problem meeting their folate needs (at least 400 mcg a day).

Nonetheless, because folate is so important for the developing fetus in the first three weeks of pregnancy, before many women realize they are pregnant, many doctors recommend that all women who could potentially become pregnant take a vitamin containing 400 mcg of folate. The best supplements also contain vitamin B$_{12}$ and do not exceed 400 mcg, because folate can mask a vitamin B$_{12}$ deficiency, and too much supplemented folate can be a problem as well. Most prenatal vitamins and multivitamins have adequate amounts of both of these nutrients. Alternatively, you may want to choose a favorite fortified breakfast cereal and eat it on most mornings. Many breakfast cereals contain a low dose of multivitamin in each serving.

Your body's requirement for vitamin B$_{12}$, needed for normal cell division and protein synthesis, is only slightly elevated during pregnancy (2.2 mcg vs. 2.0 mcg). Animal products contain B$_{12}$ from the bacteria living in their digestive tracts. As food is an unreliable source of this nutrient, a daily source of vitamin B$_{12}$, such as a

FOLATE CONTENT OF FOODS

FOOD	FOLATE CONTENT (IN MCG)
Instant oatmeal (1 package)	150
Corn flakes (1¼ cups)	100
Granola (¼ cup)	99
Asparagus (1 cup cooked)	172
Broccoli (1 cup cooked)	76
Collards (1 cup cooked)	128
Spinach (1 cup cooked)	220
Tomato juice (1 cup)	47
Orange juice (1 cup)	109
Cantaloupe (1 cup chunks)	27
Black beans (½ cup cooked)	128
Lentils (½ cup cooked)	179
Pinto beans (½ cup cooked)	147
Peanuts (2 tbsp)	35

Source: J. A. T. Pennington, *Bowes and Church's Food Values of Portions Commonly Used,* 17th ed. (Philadelphia: J. B. Lippincott, 1998).

5-mcg supplement or a serving of enriched cereal or fortified soy milk, also should be included.

Your need for vitamin D doubles during pregnancy, as it plays an important role in helping your body to absorb calcium from your foods. Oddly, unlike any of the other vitamins, your skin cells can make all the vitamin D your body needs if you simply spend fifteen minutes in the sun on most days. However, for some women this is impractical. If so, fortified food sources such as cereals, soy milks, and meat substitutes can provide plenty of vitamin D. Cow's milk is fortified, too, but it tends to tip the calcium balance scales in the wrong direction, and it is not well tolerated by many women. Vitamin D supplements are generally not recommended because even small excesses are toxic to both mother and baby and can cause fetal abnormalities. The most healthful combination is a brief walk in the sun each day and a vitamin D–fortified snack.

Most obstetricians recommend prenatal multivitamins, designed specifically to meet the nutrient needs of pregnant women. If you need a supplement, your obstetrician will help you find the right one for you.

Putting It All Together

Now you've learned how easy complete nutrition during pregnancy can be. Just remember that foods from the plant kingdom are naturally rich in the nutrients your baby needs to grow and that you need for health. All you have to do is build your meals out of grains, vegetables, legumes, and fruit, a few servings of B_{12}-fortified foods such as fortified soy milk, and perhaps a prenatal vitamin supplement.

Special Concerns

Many pregnant women experience nausea, constipation, or heartburn while pregnant. These conditions are temporary and usually can be successfully managed with a few small adjustments.

Nausea

Nausea or "morning sickness," as it is often called, is very common during the first trimester of pregnancy and can occur at any time of the day. The nausea of early pregnancy is caused by hormonal changes—especially the presence of progesterone and estrogen in the stomach. For some people, the nausea will persist throughout pregnancy, but for most women it disappears by the fourth month. For many women, an empty stomach triggers nausea, so it often occurs first thing in the morning.

Researchers at Cornell University have an explanation for the nausea associated with pregnancy. They call it "wellness insurance," because their studies show that it may be a way to protect the developing fetus from toxins and pathogens. During the first trimester of pregnancy, a mother's immune system is suppressed so that she won't reject the growing fetus. As a result, her defenses against food pathogens also are lowered. Their studies found that the foods that most commonly cause nausea are meat, fish, and eggs as well as strong and bitter-tasting vegetables such as broccoli and brussels sprouts, and bitter-tasting drinks such as coffee. Not surprisingly, meat, fish, and eggs are more likely to contain pathogens than most other foods. And many toxins have bitter tastes so an early-pregnancy aversion to bitter foods would likely be protective. These biologists also point out that in societies where meat and animal products are not consumed, morning sickness is nearly nonexistent.

Whatever the reason for it, it still needs to be managed. Many new moms are concerned that they are not eating enough to nourish their fetus during this important time. Therefore it is important to find ways to minimize the symptoms of morning sickness and to find nourishing foods that do not cause nausea.

Some mothers have success with the following strategies:

Avoid an empty stomach. Frequent small meals and nutritious snacks often help stave off nausea.

Keep food near the bed. Try eating a small amount of bland food before getting up in the morning to ward off early-morning nausea. Dry crackers or plain bread usually are a good choice.

Eat healthy foods that are well tolerated. During the first trimester, many mothers experience aversion to certain foods. Take note of the foods that you are comfortable eating and try to plan balanced meals using them. Seek out the advice of a nutritionist if you want help. On the days when you are feeling better, try to broaden your choices to include other nutrient-rich foods.

Avoid liquids with meals. If you experience nausea from drinking liquids with foods, try separating them by consuming your water or other beverages between meals.

Constipation

Many women experience constipation during pregnancy, especially in the last trimester because of the hormonal state of the body. To complicate matters, the growing fetus puts uncomfortable pressure on the intestines. In addition, iron and calcium supplements can cause constipation. For this reason, it is important not to take more of these nutrients than is necessary to meet your needs. To reduce problems with constipation, choose fiber-rich foods, do moderate exercise daily, and drink plenty of fluids. Drinking a warm beverage after a morning walk sometimes can help.

Heartburn

When you experience heartburn, you are feeling the reflux of stomach acid into the esophagus. It's common during pregnancy because the growing fetus puts pressure on the stomach, pushing acid upward. Higher levels of progesterone during pregnancy relax the valve that normally prevents that from happening.

Here are some tips that will help.

- Eat smaller, more frequent meals.
- Sit or stand for at least an hour after your meal.
- Take a brief walk after your meals.
- Avoid acidic and fatty foods as well as caffeine, carbonated beverages, chocolate, and peppermint.
- Eat slowly, and chew your food thoroughly.
- Be sure to avoid meat, dairy products, and eggs, which are often harder to digest than healthy plant foods.

Keeping Your Body Toxin-Free

The developing fetus is very small and, as such, is quite sensitive to the effects of chemicals. Whenever possible, try to avoid any and all potentially toxic substances. Some might even be hiding in foods that you thought were good for you.

Fish, for example, poses some special concerns for pregnant women. Studies at Wayne State University in 1997 showed that women who regularly ate fish, even many years before becoming pregnant, were more likely to have babies who were sluggish at birth, had small head circumferences, and had developmental problems. Fish often contains high levels of heavy metals, pesticides, and industrial chemicals such as polychlorinated biphenyls (PCBs). Fish consumption appears to affect fertility as well. Women who consume even low levels of contaminated fish have a more difficult time conceiving. Some of these chemicals remain in the body for many years.

Other meats, including beef, pork, lamb, and poultry, often contain pesticides, environmental toxins such as dioxin, and antibiotics. Pesticides are spread on feed grains, and environmental toxins occur in the soil, water, and air. Animals who consume these feed grains concentrate these toxins in their fat and muscles. If you eat chicken, for example, you could well be eating the pesticides that were spread on large numbers of plants and are now concentrated in the meat. Animals raised for meat are often fed antibiotics as growth promoters. Conventionally grown fruits and vegetables also may have pesticides on their outer surfaces. Be sure to wash your fresh produce thoroughly before eating it.

Medicines, too, that may be helpful for you may be deleterious to the developing fetus. Talk to your doctor about any and all medicines—prescription, over-the-counter, supplements, and herbal preparations—before taking them when you are pregnant.

Alcoholic beverages should never be consumed during pregnancy because alcohol can easily reach the fetus and impair fetal development. Fetal alcohol syndrome is a common problem among the children of women who drink regularly, especially during the early stages of pregnancy. This means you should avoid even occasional consumption of small amounts of alcohol. Cigarette smoking and any other use of tobacco also should be avoided during pregnancy because tobacco constricts blood flow to the baby, slowing growth, and greatly increasing the risk of having a very-low-birth-weight baby.

Remember that what you choose to eat and do during pregnancy has lifelong effects on your child's development and long-term health. Your efforts to provide your child with complete nourishment and a toxin-free environment will pay off for your child's entire life.

4

Worry-Free Breastfeeding

The Perfect Food for Babies

The ideal food for a newborn baby is mother's milk. Through her breast milk, a new mother provides the nutrients essential for an infant's development in the first months of life. Breast milk is easily digested and provides enough fluids to keep your baby from feeling thirsty or becoming constipated. And, just as important, breastfeeding creates a lasting bond between you and your baby that helps you learn your child's cues faster and provides a source of enjoyment for both of you.

Breastfeeding also protects against illness. During the first few days of lactation, mothers produce colostrum, a yellowish precursor to breast milk that is rich in antibodies that protect newborns against infection. When the breast milk comes in three or four days after birth, antibodies manufactured by the mother's immune system continue to pass to babies, helping them ward off infection for as long as they nurse. Breastfed babies are less likely than formula-fed babies to develop digestive problems, ear infections, anemia, diabetes, and other health problems.

Sucking at the breast even helps with your baby's oral development. Breastfed babies have good cheekbone development, jaw alignment, and fewer speech impediments. Therefore they are less likely to need braces or other orthodontal care later in life.

As recently as the 1960s, commercial baby formulas were considered superior to breast milk. Women who wanted to breastfeed were often talked out of it by well-meaning pediatricians. Believing they were doing what was best for their babies, most mothers followed their doctor's advice and bought expensive formula that had to be mixed with water, heated, and bottled before a hungry baby could be fed. Today physicians understand that while formula can certainly sustain newborns, it is not an exact substitute for breast milk; many of the substances that occur naturally in breast milk cannot be re-created in a commercial imitation.

Benefits for Mothers

If you choose to breastfeed, you will likely find that life is simple for your newborn as it is for most healthy infants. They let you know when they're hungry, nurse eagerly until they are satisfied, then drift off to sleep with a look of contentment on their face; it's the easiest way to keep babies happy. Breastfeeding can make life simpler for you, too. No measuring and mixing are necessary and, in most cases, no worry is needed about how much breast milk your baby is consuming.

Breastfeeding has positive effects on the mother's body as well. When your baby nurses right after birth, it causes uterine contractions that reduce bleeding and allow of the uterus to quickly regain its shape. And because producing breast milk requires a lot of energy, breastfeeding mothers burn more calories and, generally, return to their prepregnancy weight faster than bottle-feeding mothers.

How Much and How Often?

Most pediatricians believe that babies themselves are the best judges of how much to eat. Signs that a baby is getting enough to eat include gaining weight every week, urinating six to eight times a day, sleeping well, and being responsive to their mothers. Regular examinations by a pediatrician with monthly weighings will reassure parents who are watching their baby's growth.

Most pediatricians recommend feeding infants when they demand it, rather than trying to set a rigid schedule. Since breast milk is so easily digested, babies may be ready to nurse again within a short time. Generally speaking, babies want to nurse about every two hours. But each infant is different. One may be hungry an hour after the last meal, while another is content for three to four hours between feedings. Fortunate mothers who find that their babies sleep four or five hours at a stretch each night may be worried that their babies aren't eating enough. But as long as your baby is healthy and gaining weight, there is no need to urge him or her to nurse more often. Similarly, a newborn who cries every two hours all night long is perfectly normal, too, even though an exhausted mother may be amazed that a tiny infant could eat so often.

During the first weeks you may have some slight discomfort as your body adjusts. Your breasts may feel engorged and sensitive. Sticking with it through this brief period brings great rewards. Within two weeks or so your body will "know" how much milk to produce due to a remarkable physiological response of "supply and demand." The more your growing baby nurses, the more milk you'll produce.

After a few weeks, most mothers and babies will have settled into a relaxed routine. Mom will understand her infant's "language"—how baby shows when he or she is hungry, sleepy, or playful—and she will see that breastfeeding is tremendously comforting to her baby. Studies show that breastfeeding gives your infant a close bond with you and helps build a feeling of safety and security for your child.

Infants sometimes want to nurse when they are tired or grumpy, but not particularly hungry. And even though babies will have emptied both breasts after ten minutes or so of feeding, they will probably still want to nurse. Babies allowed to continue nursing until finished will feel nurtured and satisfied as well as full. Formula-fed babies and breastfed babies rushed through nursing may become fussy and suck frantically on their fists or blankets. You can take your cues from your baby. Some will turn away from the breast after a short time, while others seem to need long, comforting feedings.

Complete Nutrition for Breastfed Babies

For the first four to six months of life, babies will get the nourishment they need from breast milk and a little regular sun exposure. Infants thrive on breast milk from their mothers. Breast milk is rich in the vitamins, minerals, proteins, carbohydrates, and fats that an

Be Patient with Yourself

In the weeks before my first child's birth, I pored over books about infants and felt sure that despite my lack of experience, I could handle everything from bathing to bedtime.

The reality of caring for a baby was a bit of a shock. I was awkward with everything at first—all thumbs at diapering, frustrated when my baby stayed awake long after my own bedtime, and frightened she would slip right out of my hands in the bath. But the biggest shock was breastfeeding. None of the experts had warned that it might be uncomfortable. The first few feedings were downright painful. My tiny, seven-pound baby latched on to me with the strength of a titan, and my breasts were so engorged it hurt even to put on my bra.

After three days I told the nurse at my pediatrician's office that I needed information on formulas because I couldn't go on. "It is a bit uncomfortable at first," she said in a matter-of-fact tone, "but it does get better. Your body learns how much milk to produce. Then it's a snap."

That bit of encouragement saved me from months of mixing, measuring, and washing bottles. Within three weeks, breastfeeding was second nature. It seemed miraculous that my body made just the right amount of milk—no more, no less. My baby grew plump and healthy, and I took her everywhere, even hiking in the woods, because I didn't have to bring along a case full of bottles and formula. When she was hungry I could feed her immediately, day or night, and she was content and happy.

Since then I've told dozens of expectant women what I had never read: Be patient. The discomfort lasts only a short time, and it's followed by months of easy, convenient, and tender feedings.

KATHY GUILLERMO

infant needs. When breastfeeding mothers consume a nutrient-rich diet, their breast milk is consequently also full of nutrients, as we will see later in this chapter.

Babies, just like adults, need vitamin D, which normally comes from sunlight touching the skin, rather than from food sources. A few minutes of exposure to indirect sunlight each day, adding up to about two hours each week, will supply infants with adequate vitamin D.

The American Academy of Pediatrics, in its Breastfeeding Guidelines, states that "exclusive breast feeding is ideal nutrition and sufficient to support optimal growth and development for approximately the first six months of life." Nonetheless, in special circumstances some doctors and nutritionists recommend additional vitamins. In the United States, most babies are given a one-time dose of vitamin K at birth, because vitamin K does not reach the fetus well and is low in breast milk. Deficiencies can cause hemorrhaging and death. Infants should not receive supplemental vitamin K after that time, as large doses of the synthetic version can be toxic. For babies living where sun exposure is limited, as in cloudy climates or in the Far North or the Far South, the baby's physician may recommend a vitamin D supplement ($10 \mu g$). As you begin introducing new foods to your baby at four to six months, iron-fortified cereals are a good way to meet your baby's need for iron (1mg/kg/day). If you are not regularly consuming vitamin B_{12} from fortified food products or supplements, your baby may require a B_{12} supplement. Of course, it makes good sense for you to adjust your eating habits to include vitamin B_{12}-fortified foods so both you and your nursing baby get the benefits of this essential nutrient.

Breastfed babies generally don't need to be given water, as there is enough fluid in breast milk to keep them well hydrated. However, during very hot weather or when they have a fever, babies can benefit from extra fluids and may readily accept a bottle of water.

Milk from cows and goats is quite different in composition from human breast milk and therefore should not be fed to human infants. Human milk, which is designed specifically for promoting infant health, is much lower in protein, calcium, and sodium, and higher in mono- and polyunsaturated fats, carbohydrates, folate, and vitamin C.

If You Need a Formula

Although breastfeeding is ideal, sometimes it's impossible. If a formula must be used for health reasons, such as medication use or an infection in the mother that could pass into breast milk, or because someone other than the birth mother is caring for the baby, be assured that your baby can thrive on it. There are many different kinds of formula available. The best choice is a commercial soy formula, which is also the first choice of most hospital nurseries. It is important to use soy formula, specifically made for infants under twelve months, and not commercial soy milk, which is intended for older children and adults. Babies have special nutritional needs and require a formula designed to meet them.

COMPARING HUMAN AND ANIMAL MILKS (PER CUP)

NUTRIENT	HUMAN MILK	COW'S MILK	GOAT'S MILK
Calories	176	150	168
Protein (g)	2.4	8.0	8.7
Fat (g)	11.2	8.1	10.1
Saturated fat (g)	4.8	5.1	6.5
Monounsaturated fat (g)	4.0	2.4	2.7
Polyunsaturated fat (g)	1.6	0.3	0.4
Carbohydrate (g)	16.8	11.4	10.9
Folic acid (mcg)	16	12	1
Vitamin C (mg)	16	2	3
Sodium (mg)	40	120	122
Iron (mg)	0.08	0.12	0.12
Calcium (mg)	80	291	326

Source: J. A. T. Pennington. *Bowe and Church's Food Values of Portions Commonly Used,* 17th ed. (Philadelphia: J. B. Lippincott, 1998).

An alternative worth exploring is "breast milk banking." Hospitals in some areas may be able to provide you with human breast milk for your baby. Contact your local hospital pediatrics department or your local La Leche League, an international breastfeeding support organization, to find out more about whether breast milk banking is available in your area.

The reasons for choosing soy formula over cow's milk formula are compelling. Most food sensitivities are reactions to proteins. The proteins found in breast milk are intended for human babies (with the exception of those foreign proteins that may pass into the milk from the mother's diet). Cow's milk formula, on the other hand, contains proteins that would be tolerated by a calf but not always by a human baby. These proteins can cause respiratory problems, canker sores, skin conditions, and other sensitivities. Cow's milk also can irritate a baby's digestive tract, causing a loss of blood in the intestine and a gradual loss of iron. For these reasons pediatricians never recommend that whole cow's milk (as opposed to formula) be given to infants.

When foreign proteins enter the body, the immune system makes antibodies to them. The American Academy of Pediatrics reported that substantial evidence based on more than ninety research studies suggested that antibodies to cow's milk protein may, in some children, destroy the insulin-producing cells of the body, leading to Type I diabetes.

Establishing a Schedule

Feeding on demand doesn't mean mother must be a slave to breastfeeding, although she must always consider her baby's needs first. Most infants will settle into a routine after a few weeks, and sometime between the sixth and the twelfth week, most babies no longer want a middle-of-the-night feeding, to their parents' great relief.

Some babies, however, seem to be nocturnal. They sleep for long periods during the day and wake up only long enough to yawn, nurse, and fall asleep again. Groggy days can then mean high-energy nights. You may be startled to find your baby alert and giggling at 3:00 A.M., and ready to nurse every two hours all night long.

HUMAN MILK AND BABY FORMULAS (PER CUP)

NUTRIENT	HUMAN MILK	SOY FORMULA (PROSOBEE)	COW'S MILK FORMULA (ENFAMIL)
Calories	176	160	160
Protein (g)	2.4	4.8	3.2
Fat (g)	11.2	8.8	8.8
Saturated fat (g)	4.8	4.0	4.0
Monounsaturated fat (g)	4.0	1.6	1.6
Polyunsaturated fat (g)	1.6	2.4	2.4
Carbohydrate (g)	16.8	16.0	16.8
Folic acid (mcg)	16	24	24
Vitamin C (mg)	16	16	16
Sodium (mg)	40	56	40
Iron (mg)	0.08	3.0	0.24
Calcium (mg)	80	152	112

Source: J. A. T. Pennington. *Bowes and Church's Food Values of Portions Commonly Used,* 17th ed. (Philadelphia: J. B. Lippincott, 1998).

With a little patience it is possible to turn this lopsided schedule around. Instead of letting your baby sleep for four or five hours during the day, gently wake him or her up after three hours. Most babies will be ready to nurse after a few minutes and, eventually, will learn to wake more frequently during the day. During the night, don't rush immediately to your baby at the first whimper or sound of restlessness. Sometimes babies will waken briefly, then drift back to sleep within minutes. If they've had plenty to eat during the day and are fed just before bedtime, they will be content to sleep for longer periods between feedings at night. Keeping the lights dimmed or turned off during nighttime feedings will also help your baby go back to sleep.

Of course, if your baby doesn't go back to sleep, but begins to cry, then go ahead and feed him or her. Women who breastfeed have an advantage because they don't have to make their babies wait—and become fully awake—while they heat a bottle.

Preventing Colic

About one of five babies will suffer from colic during the first months of life. Colicky babies have gas and cry for long periods, usually in the evening, and nothing their concerned parents do seems to help. There are many theories about the causes of colic, but it is generally believed to be an irritation caused by certain foods.

A switch from cow's milk formula to breastfeeding or to a soy-based formula usually takes care of the baby's discomfort. Sometimes, however, even breastfed babies develop colic. In these cases the problem is often in their mother's diet. A report published in the journal *Pediatrics* showed that when a nursing mother eats dairy products, cow's milk proteins are passed to her baby through her breast milk. Previously it was believed that animal proteins could not end up in breast milk because they were completely broken down in the digestive tract. It is now known that surprisingly large protein molecules pass from the digestive tract into the blood and can reach the nursing baby.

A survey of 272 breastfeeding mothers showed that many babies became colicky when their mothers ate certain foods. Those most likely to cause problems were cow's milk; onions; and cruciferous vegetables such as broccoli, cauliflower, and cabbage. If your baby is colicky, simply avoid these foods during the first four months of breastfeeding.

When to Wean

Mothers often have mixed feelings about weaning. In one sense you may enjoy your baby's burgeoning self-sufficiency. On the other hand, you may miss the closeness that breastfeeding brings. As with most of the changes that occur in the first two years, there is no need to hurry; there is no "perfect" time to wean a baby. Some

Mom's Diet and Colicky Babies

Many new parents discover through trial and error how a mother's diet can affect a breastfeeding baby. I once took a train to New York to give a talk to pediatricians on children's diets. The car was nearly deserted and quiet, except for one wailing infant. His frantic parents were trying to console him but nothing seemed to help. At the risk of being intrusive, I asked the young couple if they had noticed if certain foods affected their baby's disposition. "I'm breastfeeding," the mother said, "so all he gets is breast milk. But this happens every time I have either milk, coffee, or chocolate."

NEAL BARNARD, M.D.

mothers breastfeed for a few months, then wean to formula in a bottle. Others continue to breastfeed until the child's second birthday and sometimes even later. The only hard-and-fast rule is that it's essential for babies to have breast milk or formula for at least the first year; what happens beyond that will depend on the needs of mother and baby.

Once babies are eating solid foods well, by about nine to fifteen months, the amount of breast milk or formula they consume decreases. By this age your baby may be nursing or bottle feeding three to four times a day (usually after each meal and at bedtime or between meals and at bedtime), and should be drinking water, juice, or soy formula from a cup (see chapter 5 for specifics on introducing solid foods). Your child may be less interested in nursing and easily distracted from the breast or the bottle. At this point you may want to think about weaning. Ideally this should be a gradual process, taking place over weeks or months. This gives your baby time to adjust and allows breast milk production to decrease naturally.

You can begin weaning by omitting one bottle-feeding or breastfeeding a day. It doesn't matter which one, but it will be easiest if it's the feeding your baby cares least about, perhaps in the morning or early afternoon. After a week or two, another feeding can be omitted. The same schedule can be followed for the third daily feeding and the fourth if your baby is still nursing that often. Babies between nine and twelve months should be offered soy formula in a cup with their meals. If they are older than a year and eating solid foods, it's best to give them soy or rice milk fortified with calcium and vitamin D.

It's fine to wean even more gradually. Two feedings can be eliminated at about twelve months, for example, and your baby can continue to nurse or bottle feed just once a day through the second year. This may be a good way to wean babies who find breastfeeding or their bottle so comforting that they insist on nursing long after they are happily drinking soy milk from a cup.

If you need to stop breastfeeding before six months for any reason, wean your baby to a bottle. Some babies resist bottles—the rubber nipple just isn't as soft and as warm as the mother's breast—so if possible, babies should be introduced to the bottle well before weaning. Expressing breast milk and feeding it to your baby in a bottle once or twice a week during the first months is one way to do this. You may want to accustom your baby to bottle and formula even if you plan to continue to breastfeed, as this allows you to leave their infants in someone else's care if you need to go out for several hours. You may wean from breast to bottle by substituting one bottle feeding for one breastfeeding every day for a week and so on.

Some parents discourage dependence on the bottle by not giving it to their babies at mealtimes and at bedtime. They can use a cup, with a parent's help, when they eat solid food and then have a bottle afterward or between meals. Avoid giving your child a bottle to take to bed because if your child falls asleep while drinking, the formula or juice remains in the mouth for several hours and bathes the teeth, causing tooth decay over time. Many babies find comfort in soft blankets or a stuffed toy (without small pieces that could choke infants if removed). Cuddling a favorite toy can help ease the temporary stress of losing the bottle.

Mother's Food Choices Matter

A nursing mother's diet can have a profound effect on her baby. A good rule of thumb is that whatever you eat, your baby eats, too. Healthy nutrients and contaminants alike pass from breast milk to baby. Fortunately, eating well is really quite easy. As described in chapter 1, an optimal diet is different from that followed by most people in North America and Europe, where diets tend to be fat-rich and vitamin-poor. The best diets derive their nutrients from the New Four Food Groups: vegetables (fresh or frozen), fresh fruit, legumes (beans, peas, or lentils), and whole grains. There is no need to eat fatty, sugary, and refined packaged foods nor fish, meat, eggs, and dairy products.

The question of what is a perfect diet is always controversial, especially for new mothers. However, a plant-based, or vegan, diet supplemented with vitamin B_{12} helps keep you slim and resistant to illness while providing all the nutrients necessary for optimal health. Contrary to popular belief, plant-based diets have plenty of protein to meet your needs (see chapter 3 for more details).

Babies will take a substantial amount of calcium from breast milk, so it is essential for nursing mothers to eat foods rich in this mineral. The best sources of readily absorbable calcium are in green vegetables such as broccoli, kale, collards, and mustard greens, as well as in legumes (beans, peas, and lentils). In fact, vegetables contain so many essential nutrients that they should make up at least half of your diet. Women who have difficulty digesting broccoli or other vegetables may wish to cook them longer; this does not reduce their calcium content. Avoid broccoli if your baby is colicky. Calcium-fortified foods such as orange and apple juice, tofu, soy milk, and cereals also provide plenty of calcium without dairy's disadvantages. Beans, peas, and lentils contain not only calcium but also other minerals, vitamins, fiber, protein, and small amounts of healthful fats.

Include a source of vitamin B_{12} in your daily menu, such as a serving of fortified cereal or soy milk, nutritional yeast, or any common multiple vitamin. Humans need only about 1 microgram of vitamin B_{12} per day, but since our bodies store this vitamin, it is only necessary to eat foods rich in B_{12} every day or two. Vitamin B_{12} may be listed on multivitamins or food labels by its chemical names, cobalamin or cyanocobalamin. Large doses of some vitamins may pass through breast milk and make your baby ill, however, so supplements should be discussed with a doctor first.

Nursing mothers need to drink plenty of fluids. Water, juice, and

DAILY MEAL PLANNING GUIDELINES
FOR NURSING WOMEN

Whole grains, breads, cereals: 8 or more servings Choose *whole* grains whenever possible.	Serving: 1 slice bread, ½ bun or bagel, ½ cup cooked cereal, grain, or pasta, ¾ to 1 cup ready-to-eat cereal
Legumes, nuts, seeds, nondairy milks: 6 or more servings Choose calcium-rich foods such as fortified soy milk, tofu, and beans.	Serving: ½ cup cooked beans, 4 oz tempeh or tofu, 3 oz meat analogue, 2 tbsp nuts, seeds, nut or seed butter, 1 cup fortified soy milk or other nondairy milk
Vegetables: 5 or more servings Choose at least one dark green vegetable daily. Broccoli, kale, collard greens, mustard greens, and bok choy are good calcium-rich vegetables.	Serving: ½ cup cooked or 1 cup raw
Fruits: 4 or more servings Chooose fresh fruit and calcium-fortified juices.	Serving: ½ cup canned fruit or juice or 1 medium fruit, or 1 cup fruit pieces

Source: Adapted from a Vegetarian Nutrition Dietetic Practice Group, American Dietetic Association, 1996.

other nondairy beverages such as soy milk are good choices. In addition to your usual fluid intake, nursing mothers should drink as much liquid as your baby takes from you. One way to do this is to drink a glass of water or soy milk ten to fifteen minutes before feeding your baby. Or sip from your glass while your baby nurses. It's a good idea to avoid drinking hot liquids while breastfeeding, as a sudden movement could result in an accidental scalding.

Moms can generally consume decaffeinated and herbal teas and decaffeinated coffee without causing babies any harm, though some mothers find that when they drink coffee their babies become

Healthy Vitamin B$_{12}$ Sources

- All common multivitamins
- Fortified cereals such as Kellogg's Corn Flakes, Total, and Product 19
- Fortified soy milk
- Red Star nutritional yeast

fussy (see "Preventing Colic" page 49). Since alcohol will pass through to breast milk, it is best to avoid it while nursing.

A diet built from a variety of vegetables, fruits, grains, and legumes, along with a source of vitamin B$_{12}$, is satisfying and healthy. Combined with simple exercise, such as brisk walking several days a week, and plenty of rest, it will help new mothers feel fit and energetic. Getting sufficient rest is important and likely will be a challenge in the first weeks. Although breastfeeding is the easiest way to feed newborns, producing milk requires the body to work. If you get overtired you may find that your milk supply decreases, and suddenly your baby is demanding to be fed every hour. Napping, or at least resting when baby naps, will help.

A Clean Food Supply for Your Baby

A plant-based, or vegan, diet has the added advantage of reducing the levels of environmental contaminants in breast milk. Studies show that women who consume meat have higher levels of chemical contaminants in their breast milk, probably because these chemicals tend to concentrate in animal tissues. Plant foods have much lower levels of contaminants than foods from animal sources, and are even cleaner when they are grown organically.

Fish, touted as a good alternative to red meat, is often very high in contaminants. Fish commonly contain mercury, polychlorinated biphenyls (PCBs), and other organochlorine pesticides, which can pass through breast milk to nursing babies. These contaminants, which have been linked to cancer and other health problems, tend to accumulate in body fat and remain in the body for decades. A breastfeeding mother can easily pass half of her accumulated load of certain organochlorines to her baby.

Dairy products, including cow's milk, raise this same contamination concern. Since pesticides and other contaminants tend to concentrate in milk, nursing mothers who eat dairy products pass them along to their babies. Cow's milk proteins also can enter breast milk. As discussed above, these proteins can cause colic, as well as contributing to allergic reactions, and a whole host of problems in babies.

Caring for a newborn child is an exciting, rewarding, and at times exhausting experience for most parents. As a parent you have accomplished the amazing feat of giving life to a new person. You now have the opportunity to offer your baby love and care as well as the gift of good health. Do yourself and your baby a lifelong favor by choosing a clean, safe, healthy, and delicious vegetarian diet while breastfeeding.

Nursing the World Back to Health

Breastfeeding not only benefits mother and child but also has some advantages you might not have imagined. The ultimate in renewable resources, human milk arrives in the breast as a baby is born and is supplied in just the right amount for as long as the mother and the baby want it to be. It's practically free, it provides optimal nutrition, is clean and sterile, and protects the baby from a variety of ailments.

- In one study, a group of infants fed artificial milk for six months had sixteen times greater health care costs than breastfed infants.

- Worldwide, breastfeeding helps to curb overpopulation, mostly because lactation slows the return of menses after birth. In some countries, breastfeeding prevents an average of four to six births per woman.

- Formula production requires much higher use of natural resources such as land and water and causes more pollution than breast milk production.

LA LECHE LEAGUE

5

The Transition
to Solid Foods

The introduction of solid foods is an exciting new step in a baby's development. Different tastes and textures enchant some infants, while others resist the "foreign" substances their parents are spooning into their mouths. There are plenty of rewards and pitfalls during this time of rapid growth, and this chapter will guide you through them.

Most pediatricians recommend introducing solids between four and six months. By this time your baby may be quite interested in what other family members are doing at the dinner table, and may even try to grab the utensil from your hand. Although babies don't need table food yet, their natural inclination is to imitate their parents.

Babies don't actually derive much nourishment from solids for the first few weeks as they learn how to accept food from a spoon. Initially the natural tongue-thrust reflex will cause babies to push the food back out of their mouths as soon as the feeder puts it in. It may take several days of scraping food off your child's chin and putting it back in before he or she learns how to manipulate food with the tongue and swallow it. But there is no need to worry. Your baby is simply trying to figure out what solid food is all about and will still be getting plenty of nutrients from breast milk or soy formula.

How to Begin

One feeding of solid food a day is enough in the beginning. The time of day is less important than your baby's mood. You'll want to keep this new experience positive, so choose a time when your baby is wide awake, not overly hungry, and eager to interact with you. Whether in the morning, afternoon, or early evening, the first feeding of solid food should be an hour or more after the last breast-feeding and well before the next nap. Babies who are still full from their last meal will not be interested in eating more, and cranky babies in need of sleep won't have the patience to try this strange new practice. A comfortable position also will help. Some parents find that an infant seat works well; others prefer a high chair, with rolled towels tucked around their baby for support.

Most babies don't eat much at first, perhaps no more than a tea-spoonful. A demitasse or infant spoon with just a pea-size bite of food on it works well. For several days your baby will just taste food. After a few weeks, as toddlers learn how satisfying new foods can be, they will happily eat several teaspoonfuls.

You may prefer a commercial infant cereal as a first food, because it can be mixed with breast milk or soy formula so that your baby's first taste of solid food isn't completely foreign. Cereals made especially for babies are convenient because they are pre-cooked and ready to mix, heat, and serve in just a few minutes. Rice, corn, oats, or barley cereals are good choices. Wheat is more frequently allergenic to babies and should not be introduced before the sixth or the seventh month; some pediatricians recommend waiting until after the first birthday. For the first few weeks, cereals should be thinned with enough breast milk, soy formula, or water to be quite soupy. Cereal that is too thick and lumpy is more difficult for babies to swallow.

Commercial cereals have the advantage of being fortified with iron, but regular oatmeal and other cooked cereals can be used, too.

Grinding them with a hand food mill will make them fine enough to prevent choking.

Beyond Cereal

After a couple of weeks of feeding cereal once a day, you can introduce fruit or vegetables. Most babies are immediately drawn to the naturally sweet flavor of apples, pears, apricots, prunes, and peaches. An interest in sweet-tasting foods and a dislike of bitter-tasting ones is natural and, in fact, is genetically programmed into babies and small children. As children grow older, their tastes shift to accept a greater variety.

Fruit offered to your baby should be stewed and strained to a creamy consistency. Very ripe bananas can be mashed and mixed with a little breast milk or soy formula. If you use commercial baby food, choose one with no added sugar. It's best not to feed your baby directly from the jar unless you are going to finish the food in that sitting, because bacteria from your child's saliva will quickly spoil the remaining food.

Most babies enjoy diluted fruit juice. White grape or apple juice mixed with an equal portion of water can be given in a bottle or, for

APPROXIMATE AGE FOR INTRODUCTION OF FOODS

Birth to 6 months	4 to 6 months	6 to 7 months	7 to 8 months	8 to 9 months	10 to 12 months
breast milk or infant formula					
	iron-fortified infant cereal (not wheat-based)				
		mashed or pureed fruits and vegetables			
			legumes (i.e., lentils, peas, beans, tofu) wheat-based foods		
				juice from a cup soft finger foods	
					soft, chopped fruits and vegetables

babies at least six months old, in a cup. Holding the cup and offering tiny sips, with a pause between swallows, will help your baby learn to drink in this new way. Expect a few spills while he or she learns this skill. Because of their high sugar content, commercial juices should not be given too frequently—perhaps two or three times a week. Also, be aware that a bottle labeled "fruit juice" may contain as little as 5 percent juice. Check the labels.

While your baby is consuming mostly liquid foods—breast milk or soy formula, watered-down cereals, fruits, and juices—giving water is generally not necessary unless the weather is particularly hot. As your baby begins to eat more solid foods and is weaned off breast milk or formula, it will be important to make sure that he or she is drinking enough water and other fluids.

Some fruits, such as strained apricots and prunes, may cause loose stools. If this occurs, omit these fruits from the diet until your baby is a few months older, and give other fruit less frequently, perhaps every other day in the first weeks when he or she is still eating only one solid meal a day. Conversely, prunes, apricots, or a little diluted prune juice will act as natural laxatives for babies who become constipated. The roughage in fruit helps them stay regular.

Like fruit, fresh or frozen vegetables should be cooked and strained before being offered to your baby for the first time. For convenience, commercial baby foods without added salt or sugar may be used. Since vegetables lack the sweetness of fruit, some babies don't take to vegetables as readily as they do to fruits, but they usually grow to like them after several feedings. Sweet potatoes, carrots, squash, peas, beets, and string beans are good first choices; they lack the bitterness of broccoli, cabbage, cauliflower, turnips, kale, and other greens. You may want to add fruit juice to these stronger-tasting vegetables to make them more appealing.

Beets and green vegetables may turn the stools red and green, respectively, and some vegetables may darken the urine as well. This discoloration is harmless. Pediatricians will often recommend against feeding spinach until after the first birthday, as it can cause chapping of the lips and the anus in some babies. If certain vegetables cause loose stools or gas, they should be given less frequently or omitted from the diet until the baby is a few months older.

Even in these early months, babies can—and usually do—show

their likes and dislikes. They may prefer some foods and repeatedly refuse others. But there is no need to worry if they don't like some vegetables. It's better to feed them the vegetables they do enjoy and reintroduce the others later.

Legumes—beans, peas, tofu, and lentils—may be added to the diet after cereals, fruits, and vegetables. Lentils, chickpeas, pink beans, and kidney beans are good first choices, as they are easily prepared and are good sources of iron as well as protein. They must always be well cooked and thoroughly mashed. Soft or silken tofu is a favorite of many babies, who seem to like its texture. Mixing tofu with pureed fruits or vegetables gives it a bit more flavor.

If your baby doesn't seem comfortable with solids yet, there is no need to rush. Breast milk or soy formula should remain the main source of calories in the first six to eight months. Parents who push solid foods too enthusiastically may find that their infants don't enjoy mealtime and may even be too full to take in the amount of breast milk they need.

Adding More Foods

By six or seven months, babies look forward to solids, and may wave their arms and coo excitedly when they see Mother or Father approach with a dish of cereal or strained fruit. If they are also comfortable with a spoon, this is a good time to increase the amount of solids by adding another meal.

If your baby normally eats breakfast, a dinner or late-afternoon meal can be added. If he or she already eats dinner, you might add breakfast. Some parents like their baby to eat with the rest of the family; others find it's easier to feed the little one before the family sits down for their regular meals. Babies often have their own ideas about when to eat. They may be hungry for solids in the morning and afternoon hours, for example, and more interested in nursing in the evenings. There are no hard-and-fast rules. As long as the two meals are not too close together, it doesn't matter what time of day is chosen.

Babies usually let parents know when they are ready to add a third meal. Typically this happens sometime between the eighth and the twelfth months, but it may be sooner. Babies who readily eat two meals a day and still nurse or take soy formula four times a day are probably ready for another solid meal.

Finger Foods

As they increase the amount of solids they consume, babies also become more proficient at eating. They are curious about the foods given to them, often putting their fingers in their mouths or in the bowl if their mothers will let them, to feel the cereal, vegetables, or fruit. By six or seven months most babies are ready to try feeding themselves a few finger foods. A good first finger food is a wedge of toasted whole wheat or oat bread or a small chunk of well-cooked sweet potato, which they will gum and soften with their saliva and might smear on their faces and in their hair. Eventually they might swallow some of it. (As some babies are sensitive to wheat, it should not be a big part of the diet for the first year, as noted above.)

As your baby's manual dexterity improves, slices of soft banana, chunks of soft tofu or avocado, and beans that are cooked until quite soft and then slightly mashed are other good finger foods. If they can manage them, babies love well-cooked noodles such as rice or whole-wheat noodles once or twice a week. These should be boiled until they are very soft and then cut into short, manageable lengths. Soft-cooked vegetables such as squash (peeled with seeds removed), potatoes, and carrots are also good choices.

Learning to pick up soft chunks of food and get them into the mouth without dropping them along the way can be a laborious process for your hungry baby, so continue to offer strained foods as well. A serving of familiar food, without lumps, will keep the tummy full until the tiny fingers become adept at handling chunkier foods.

Most babies love feeding themselves and will happily squeeze vegetables between their thumbs and forefingers and anywhere else they can smear them. The mess babies make while they eat is a natural part of this process. Your child is exploring foods as well as learning how to eat them. Keeping mealtimes relaxed without too much fussing and wiping up encourages your baby to try new foods. A quick bath after mealtime will take care of any dribbles.

Gagging and Choking

Nearly toothless babies are bound to gag a bit as they learn to "gum" chunky, soft solid foods. This is rarely cause for concern, because they usually cough the problem food right back up. However, if they are frequently gagging and choking, it may be a sign that they are not yet ready for solid food.

If your baby seems to be choking but is still breathing and coughing, the best thing to do is to let them work the food out on their own. Coughing is the body's way of trying to dislodge the stuck food. Do not hit a child's back or turn him or her upside down, as these methods may actually make the problem worse. If your baby doesn't cough the food back up and is not breathing or is turning blue, put the baby on your lap sitting up with his or her back against your abdomen, or place the baby face up on his or her back, on a flat, firm surface such as a table or the floor. Place the middle and index fingers of both your hands on the midline below the rib cage and above the navel. Press gently into the child's abdomen with a quick upward thrust. Start gently and increase the pressure as needed. Repeat until the choking object is expelled. Performing the Heimlich maneuver in this way is the safest way to dislodge the choking object and help your child to begin breathing normally again.

To lessen the chance of choking, it's best not to give foods that are difficult to chew or that have skins and hulls, such as berries with seeds, whole blueberries, whole grapes (even if they are cut or mashed), raw carrot slices, peanut butter, whole corn kernels, and—for safety and health reasons—chunks of meat, peanuts, and candy.

Choosing Healthy Foods

Most babies learn to like the foods that are given to them and enjoy the flavors of simple foods that may seem bland to some adults. Parents who feed their babies from the New Four Food Groups—vegetables, grains, fruits, and legumes—do their children a favor by introducing tastes for foods that can keep them healthy later in life. Shown in the following table, the foods represented in the New Four Food Groups are the best foods for the long-term health of both children and adults (see chapter 1 for more detailed information.)

This may be a departure for some parents. For decades many people, particularly in Western cultures, have used meat and dairy products as staples of the diet. Babies and toddlers, however, have no preconceived notions and will readily take to healthy diets if their parents offer them. It's a good idea for you to base all of your family's meals on the New Four Food Groups to stay healthy and set a good example for your baby.

Eating habits we learn in childhood can stay with us throughout life. Babies who acquire a taste for excessive salt may, in later years, have problems with high blood pressure. Too many fried foods and processed sweets, with their high calorie content, may lead to obesity. Meats, chicken, fish, and dairy products, which are often laden with cholesterol and saturated fats, are best avoided altogether. Babies and adults can easily derive the nourishment they need from the New Four Food Groups, so there is no need to introduce foods that are likely to cause serious health problems later in life.

Population studies show that countries in which meat, egg, and dairy consumption is low enjoy a correspondingly low incidence of heart disease, high blood pressure, and many kinds of cancers. The opposite is true in North America and European countries where meat and dairy are served at nearly every meal and where children as young as three or four have early artery changes, called fatty streaks, that are the first step toward clogging of the arteries. In the United

---

THE NEW FOUR FOOD GROUPS

Vegetables	Carrots, sweet potatoes, green beans, broccoli, asparagus, mushrooms, cooked greens, potatoes, squash, etc.
Fruits	Apples, bananas, peaches, pears, melons, oranges, mangoes, etc.
Legumes	Beans, peas, lentils, soy milk, tofu, etc.
Whole grains	Brown rice, whole grain bread and pasta, oatmeal, corn, barley, etc.

States, cholesterol screenings are now recommended for children beginning at age three. These would be largely unnecessary if children were raised on the healthy foods recommended in this book.

In addition to laying the groundwork for chronic diseases, meats and eggs pose another serious and more immediate threat. They often harbor bacteria that can cause very serious infections. Animal products are often contaminated during the slaughter process with bacteria such as *E. coli, camphylobacter, or salmonella,* which come from the intestinal tract (i.e., feces) of animals. Since bacteria can't be seen, it's impossible to know how extensively these germs taint the meat at your grocery store.

An increasingly common contaminant of meat, a particularly dangerous strain of bacteria, *E. coli* O157:H7, may cause nausea, vomiting, and severe diarrhea if consumed by adults, mimicking a "stomach flu." But babies and young children, with their immature immune systems, are at much greater risk. Recent outbreaks of *E. coli* poisoning from contaminated meat have been responsible for numerous deaths among children. Other infectious bacteria, especially *salmonella* and *camphylobacter,* are now found—still alive—in about two-thirds of chicken products in grocery stores. Undercooked eggs that contain *salmonella* frequently pass this infection to babies. These bacteria can easily contaminate anything eggs or meat come in contact with—utensils, food preparation surfaces, towels, sponges, even the food preparer's hands. Some of these germs can occasionally be found on the surfaces of fruits and vegetables, especially if the produce has come in contact with meat, so to be safe, wash produce before serving it to children.

For all of these reasons—cholesterol, fat, infectious bacteria, and many others—it is best to help your baby steer clear of meats and other animal products and to grow up on healthy whole grains, vegetables, fruits, and legumes.

Supplements for a Growing Baby

Babies who are eating solids from the New Four Food Groups, as well as nursing or taking soy formula, should be given a vitamin B_{12} supplement. Vitamin B_{12} is essential for healthy nerves and healthy blood. A tiny daily intake—0.5 microgram—is all that is needed, because our bodies store it well. Vitamin B_{12} is included in typical children's multivitamins. B_{12} is also found in foods from animal sources because the bacteria in their gastrointestinal tracts manufacture it. However, the health risks associated with meat and dairy products are such that it is better to take B_{12} in another form.

Vitamin D is important for strong bones, among other functions in the body. Inadequate amounts can result in soft bones and improper physical development. As discussed in chapter 3, babies' bodies manufacture vitamin D if they are exposed to adequate sunshine for about twenty minutes a day on average. Be sure to apply suncreen if your child is in the sun for longer periods of time. If sun exposure isn't possible because of the climate, or if the baby's skin is dark, breastfed babies should be given a vitamin D supplement of 400 IU (international units). Soy formula is usually fortified with vitamin D, so formula-fed babies will not need a supplement until they go off formula.

Similarly, soy formulas are often fortified with iron to prevent anemia, which sometimes occurs in infants over four months of age. Breastfeeding mothers who eat a varied, healthy diet can supply their babies with adequate iron through breast milk. Although pediatricians once recommended that babies be given hard-cooked, mashed egg yolks to supply iron, we now know that egg yolks can inhibit the body's absorption of iron from other sources. The best sources of iron are found in lentils, beans, vegetables, and fortified cereals.

In the past decade, pediatricians have begun recommending fluoride for babies older than six months. Fluoride helps strengthen babies' teeth and reduces the likelihood that children will develop cavities in later years, particularly if good dental hygiene is also practiced. If fluoride is added to the water supply and the water is good in your area, there is no need for this supplement as long as water is given in a cup or a bottle or is mixed with powdered soy formula.

Diet by the First Birthday

The first year is full of milestones. Your baby will learn to roll over, sit up without assistance, eat solid food, and perhaps stand or toddle about the house. If luck is with you, your baby may even sleep through the night. In the second half of their first year, babies can grasp tiny bites of food and put them in their mouths without help from Mom or Dad. Indeed, "grown up" food is very important to a one-year-old, who is relying less and less on breast milk and increasingly on solids to meet caloric needs.

Parents may worry during this time that their baby is not getting enough to eat or isn't eating enough of the right kinds of food. All babies are individuals, so what is normal for one may not be right for another. Parents may notice, for example, that the strapping baby boy who lives next door seems to be eating constantly and always has a cracker or a slice of banana in his chubby fist. By contrast, their also healthy son eats only at mealtimes, and then not very much. As long as your baby is gaining about a pound a month in the second half of the first year (all babies should have their weights checked during regular visits to a pediatrician), there is no need to worry.

Babies' appetites can be affected by teething; the tingling and discomfort in their gums may make chewing painful. Or they may be really hungry only every other day, and content with only small meals on the days in between. Babies who temporarily lose interest in food should not have it forced on them. Unless they are sick, their appetites usually pick up within a day or so. On the other hand,

Foods for a One-Year-Old

Vegetables.   Well-cooked and slightly mashed sweet potato, carrot, squash (peeled, seeds removed), broccoli, green beans, white potato (peeled), beet, ripe avocado

Fruits.   Ripe, soft, sliced banana, peach, pear, mango, cantaloupe, watermelon, scraped apple, stewed or canned fruit

Grains.   Oatmeal, cream of rice, cream of wheat; whole wheat toast, well-cooked brown rice, barley, well-cooked pasta

Legumes.   Well-cooked, lightly mashed lentils, peas, beans, including pink, black, lima, Great Northern, kidney, chickpeas, etc., soft tofu

Nursing or soy formula.   Four times daily

Be sure to include a vitamin B_{12}-fortified food or a vitamin containing this important nutrient as well.

Sample Menu for a One-Year-Old

Breakfast.   Oatmeal or other grain cereal, toast, and fresh fruit such as scraped apple or banana slices

Lunch.   Well-cooked green or yellow vegetables, whole wheat bread with a smooth nut butter thinned with soy formula

Supper.   Potatoes or well-cooked rice, legumes, fruit, and a vegetable

Plus four or more servings of soy formula or breast milk.

if your baby refuses to eat for more than one day or seems ill, consult your physician. Generally, by the end of the first year a healthy baby will be eating three meals a day and nursing or taking a soy formula bottle about four times a day.

Drinks

Babies usually like a beverage with their meals and, by their first birthdays, many drink well from a cup held by Mom or Dad. Some can even handle their own cups. If you give your child fruit juices, they should be 100 percent juice without added sugars or syrups. Juices are naturally sweet; they don't need extra sweeteners. Most pediatricians recommend limiting juices to 4 to 8 ounces a day or less, as some babies will fill up on juices and be less interested in solid foods. Since fruit juices often have a strong flavor, some babies prefer them diluted with water.

Orange juice should not be given until babies are at least nine months to one year old because their immature digestive systems are frequently upset by citrus fruits. When orange juice is introduced, it should be mixed with equal parts water for several months. If desired, the amount of water can then be gradually decreased.

Benefits of Soy and Rice Milks

For many years pediatricians encouraged mothers to introduce their babies to whole cow's milk at twelve months, usually as a first step toward weaning from the breast or from commercial formula. The emergence of health concerns about cow's milk products and the widespread availability of soy and rice milks in stores has changed this recommendation. These plant-based milks may be used in the same way as cow's milk—for drinking, on cereals, for baking, etc.

Commercially produced soy and rice milks, fortified with vitamin D and calcium, are better choices for year-old babies than cow's milk. Young children are less likely to develop allergies to these products than to cow's milk, and the problems caused by animal proteins, cholesterol, and saturated fat can be avoided. For example, the proteins in cow's milk have been connected with the Type 1 diabetes. Some children's immune systems make antibodies to the proteins in cow's milk, and these antibodies can attack and destroy the insulin-producing cells of the pancreas. Feeding nondairy milks avoids this potential problem.

Another, more immediate difficulty with cow's milk products is that they can interfere with iron balance. Researchers from the University of Iowa reported in 1990 in the *Journal of Pediatrics* that "a large proportion of babies" who are fed whole cow's milk are prone to serious iron deficiency, as milk can cause subtle intestinal bleeding. This problem may not entirely disappear after twelve months of age, and unmodified cow's milk can continue to irritate the digestive tract and cause gradual blood loss.

Over time this loss of blood cells reduces the body's store of iron. To make matters worse, when dairy products are consumed with a meal, the body becomes less efficient at absorbing iron. A cup of milk served with breakfast, lunch, or dinner will reduce the amount of iron absorbed by about half.

Adults and other children in the family may also wish to try soy or rice milk in place of cow's milk. The transition is not difficult—just as the taste buds can adjust from whole milk to reduced-fat milk in a week or two, the change to soy or rice milk is usually quick and easy. Every brand tastes different, so try several until you find the family favorite. Family members will derive the same health benefits as babies and set a good example for the youngest family member.

Adding solid foods brings your baby a step closer to being grown up. Babies are fascinated with the new tastes and enjoy gaining the independence of beginning to feed themselves. It also brings you farther along in your family's exploration of healthy foods, and how they fit into each stage of life.

DISADVANTAGES OF COW'S MILK

Cow's milk protein	● Proteins in cow's milk have been implicated in insulin-dependent diabetes.
	● Cow's milk proteins are a common cause of food allergies in children.
Cow's milk fat	● Cow's milk contains significant amounts of saturated fat (except skim products) and cholesterol that contribute to heart disease and cancer.
	● Cow's milk is low in essential fatty acids.
Cow's milk sugar	● Many older children, especially those of Asian and African ancestry, cannot digest the cow's milk sugar, lactose. The results are diarrhea and gas.
	● Galactose, one of the components of lactose, has been implicated in ovarian cancer and cataracts.
Low in iron	● Cow's milk is very low in iron and is associated with iron deficiency anemia.
	● Cow's milk causes blood loss from the intestinal tract, which reduces iron stores.
Contaminants	● Traces of antibiotics fed to cows can show up in cow's milk products.
	● Pesticides and other drugs are also frequent contaminants of dairy products.
	● Cow's milk is fortified with vitamin D. Recent studies have shown that some milk samples have an excess of vitamin D, which can be toxic.
IGF-1	● Cow's milk consumption increases the levels of insulinlike growth factor (IGF-1) in the blood of individuals who regularly consume cow's milk.
	● Higher levels of IGF-1 are linked to cancer of the breast and prostate.

6

Feeding Toddlers

Babies make tremendous progress during the first eighteen to twenty-four months of life. They go from helpless newborns relying on their parents for their every need and comfort to expressive individuals determined to show Mom and Dad just how independent they can be. Speech becomes important. Toddlers both understand others and begin to experiment with words themselves—often to tell parents "No!" By age two many of your child's likes and dislikes will be fairly well established, particularly when it comes to food. Fortunately most toddlers are still curious about the new items that appear on their plates, and usually they're willing to touch, sniff, and then taste something they've never seen before.

It's Easy to Get Complete Nutrition

It's surprisingly easy to offer your child health-giving meals that provide the nourishment they need. Start out with some type of whole grain cereal or bread at each feeding and add small servings of well-cooked or grated fresh vegetables, well-cooked legumes, nondairy milk, and fresh fruit. Here is a guide to specific amounts.

DAILY MEAL PLANNING
FOR TODDLERS (1–4 YEARS)

Whole grains, breads, cereals: 4 servings

Serving: 1 slice bread, $\frac{1}{2}$ bun or bagel, $\frac{1}{2}$ cup cooked cereal, grain, or pasta, $\frac{3}{4}$ to 1 cup ready-to-eat cereal, crackers.

Choose whole grains whenever possible.

Vegetables: 2–4 tablespoons dark green vegetables, $\frac{1}{4}$ to $\frac{1}{2}$ cup other vegetables

Dark green vegetables: broccoli, kale, collard greens, mustard greens, and bok choy are good choices.

Other vegetables: any and all, fresh or frozen, raw or cooked.

Legumes, nuts, seeds, milks: $\frac{1}{4}$ to $\frac{1}{2}$ cup legumes, 3 servings breast milk, soy formula, soy milk, or other nondairy milk

Legumes: beans, peas, tofu, and lentils cooked until soft. Serving nondairy milk: 1 cup. Nuts and seeds: optional in small amounts (1–2 tbsp).

Fruits: $\frac{3}{4}$ to $1\frac{1}{2}$ cups

Fruits: any and all, fresh or frozen, raw or cooked.

Add a source of vitamin B_{12}, such as any typical children's multivitamin or vitamin-fortified cereals or soy milk, and you've covered the nutritional bases.

A Closer Look at Your Baby's Food

By the time most babies reach their first birthday, they have already been introduced to many of the foods that will be staples of a healthy diet for childhood and adulthood. Your child probably enjoys cereals, sliced bananas and other fruit, mashed beans, tofu (made from soybeans), squash, green beans, and several different kinds of vegetables. Now is a good time to broaden the variety of the foods you offer to your child.

The Whole Grain Group

Brown and white rice, millet, barley, whole wheat, buckwheat, oat-meal—there are an astonishing variety of grains. Used for many foods, including breads, pasta, pancakes, cereals, and soups, versatile grains can be flavored and prepared in many different ways. Within the pasta category, for example, there are soba noodles, spaghetti, fettuccine, lo mein noodles, and many others. Rice can be made into cakes, noodles, sweet desserts, pilafs, stir-frys, curries, "milk," and cereal. The possibilities are endless.

Most toddlers particularly enjoy grains, as they are filling and their mild flavor is appealing. And slurping a spaghetti noodle is a favorite toddler activity. Soups, sandwiches, pancakes, homemade low-fat baked goods, soy cheese pizza, and rice pudding are popular grain-based foods for young children. For example, a thick, tomato-based soup with pink beans, whole wheat noodles, and carrot chunks is nutritious and appealing to toddlers, as are sandwiches with peanut butter and banana or mini-pita pockets with grated vegetables and bean dip.

The Vegetable Group

Toddlers usually enjoy the same vegetables they were introduced to as infants. Now they're ready to move from strained to well-cooked, bite-sized chunks. Vegetables can be steamed, baked, or served raw. Toddler favorites include mashed potatoes, peas, green beans, beets and carrots, chunks of well-cooked yam, and the mild flavor of seeded yellow squash.

Some of the vegetables given to toddlers should be served raw and some should be served cooked. The longer vegetables are cooked, the more vitamins they lose, but the more digestible they become. A quick stir-fry in a hot wok with a little water will preserve much of the vitamin content, but fresh raw vegetables still are the best source of the water-soluble vitamins such as folate. On the other hand, some foods, such as broccoli and corn, are hard to digest unless they are well cooked.

And some firm vegetables can be a challenge for toddlers. Until they have their molars, chewing a crisp carrot is impossible. Even with most of their baby teeth, they are at risk of choking on a hard chunk of raw vegetable. You can get around this by washing and peeling vegetables, then slicing them into very thin strips, or by scraping them with a potato peeler or a knife. This works well with carrots, cucumbers, and green peppers. Raw, scraped vegetables can be served plain or mixed with a little applesauce. Some children who won't look at a plain carrot will happily eat a scraped carrot if it's mixed with a little nut butter and spread on a piece of whole grain bread. Peeled, seeded tomatoes, cut into chunks, are easily eaten, too.

The Legume Group

Well-cooked and slightly squashed beans are a popular finger food with toddlers. There are dozens of varieties. Among beans, for example, there are black beans, kidney beans, navy beans, chickpeas, and many others. Soybeans are used to make tofu, which, given the chance, many toddlers love. Then there are snow peas, yellow peas, and lentils, which can be turned into mouth-watering soups and stews.

As their menus broaden, toddlers will enjoy baked beans on whole wheat toast; thick lentil, potato, and carrot stew; sandwich spreads made from black beans and mild spices; and other healthy dishes. Hummus, a spread made of chickpeas, sesame tahini, and spices, can be made in a food processor or can be purchased in grocery stores. It makes a good sandwich spread or dip for raw carrot strips.

Also included in the legume group for meal-planning purposes are nondairy milks, nuts, and seeds. Nondairy milks are a good source of nutrients for small children. In the early toddler years your child may still be having some breast milk or soy formula. After weaning, soy milk and other nondairy milks made from grains such as rice or oats, fortified with calcium, vitamin B_{12}, and vitamin D, can be easily incorporated into your child's daily menu. Nuts and seeds, while high in fat, are good sources of minerals such as zinc and manganese, and can add variety to your toddler's meals.

The Fruit Group

Cooked or stewed fruits such as applesauce or baked pears are easily eaten and digested. Fruits served raw, such as sliced kiwis, bananas, melons, or mangoes, are delicious with a sandwich or as a topping for hot cereal. As with firm vegetables, crisper fruits such as apples can be scraped. Grapes and whole berries are choking hazards and should not be given until at least the third year. Baked into cakes, quick breads, or tarts, fruits add moisture and sweetness and can replace sugar and eggs in most recipes. Softer fruits such as strawberries, cantaloupes, bananas, and mangoes, can be whizzed in a blender with a little soy milk to make fruit "shakes." However they are served, fruits are important for toddlers. Like vegetables, they contain many different vitamins, complex carbohydrates, and fiber.

Children who are given fruits rather than sugary candy or other sweets will enjoy the sweet taste without giving a thought to vitamins, antioxidants, and fiber. And they will learn to choose foods that will help keep their body's weight in check as the years go by. This is rarely a concern for toddlers, who need concentrated calories to develop, but it is an increasing problem for children over age three. Toddlers who are regularly given candies and cakes will choose these "empty" calories over more healthful foods.

A wide variety of selections from the New Four Food Groups can be cooked into nutritious, filling dishes that will satisfy an active toddler (for recipe ideas, see chapter 18). Experimenting with new combinations of fresh, whole foods is an enjoyable way to provide your family, even the smallest member, with healthy, delicious meals.

If Your Toddler Won't Eat Vegetables

Toddlers are unpredictable eaters. The eighteen-month-old who loved boiled sweet potatoes last week may inexplicably refuse them this week. A two-year-old may demand celery slices every day for a month and then, one day, suddenly fling them across the dining table in disgust. Some toddlers refuse to try any vegetables for weeks on end.

Like many parents, you may be concerned that your child is not getting enough nutrients. But demanding that a strong-willed toddler finish every bit of vegetable on the plate can actually make the situation worse. Even with the best intentions, your worry about adequate nutrition can turn into a battle over who is in control. The toddler years are times of great discovery and independence, and your child, in his or her quest for ever greater autonomy, will often choose to grapple over the very issues that most concern you.

It's better not to make a fuss. Just continue to offer whatever vegetables your child will eat as well as plenty of fruits, grains, beans, and lentils. Or try mincing broccoli, green peppers, and leafy greens in a food processor and adding them to spaghetti sauce or even applesauce, as children don't know that spinach and applesauce aren't supposed to be eaten together. It's reassuring to note that fruits and vegetables share many of the same vitamins and minerals, and both have abundant fiber. Most toddlers who temporarily shun vegetables will happily eat plenty of fruit. And eventually they'll begin to eat vegetables again. In the meantime, a multivitamin formulated for toddlers will supply what's missing. However, be sure that your child is not ill. Any toddler who refuses to eat most foods or rarely seems hungry should be seen by a pediatrician.

This is a time for exercising great flexibility in your relationship with your child. Serve whatever nutritious foods they will eat, hiding foods they don't like under foods they do like. Remember that nearly every phase passes and that the vast majority of kids and parents look back on this time with wonder.

Drinks for Toddlers

Toddlers should be offered fresh water every day. And vitamin- and calcium-fortified soy and rice milk are good sources of nutrients often enjoyed by young children. Your toddler also may enjoy vegetable juices, although these should not take the place of whole vegetables. A limited amount of fruit juice without added sugar also may be offered. The amount should be limited to less than 12 ounces (1½ cups) per day, because research has shown that daily intake of larger amounts can contribute to obesity and short stature in young children.

Mothers who choose to breastfeed their babies through the second year will probably find that their toddlers are content with one to three feedings a day. Most of their calories will now come from solid food.

Toddlers and Sweets

Rich, sugary foods such as cakes and cookies may satisfy a toddler's hunger temporarily, but because they lack vitamins, fiber, and minerals, they have little or no nutritional value. Children who consume sweets regularly are displacing healthier foods with "empty" calories. Sweets also can promote tooth decay if they are eaten too often. There is no need for them. Most toddlers love the natural sweetness of fruit. They enjoy a chunk of orange or a slice of apple as much as their parents love cake or other dessert. Left to themselves, toddlers seem to prefer to satisfy their sweet tooth in healthy ways.

Encouraging Healthy Eating

If possible, meals should be relaxed times when families gather to share nutritious food. It isn't always easy to accomplish this, particularly with an active and vocal toddler. Still, parents who set a good example by eating balanced meals from the New Four Food Groups offer their young children a great gift: the opportunity to learn, right from the start, how to use foods to maintain health.

If Your Extended Family Doesn't Understand Good Nutrition

In many cultures the world over, choosing foods entirely, or almost entirely, from the New Four Food Groups has been standard practice for centuries. To others it may sound unusual. Sometimes parents embrace a healthy plant-based diet for themselves and their children, only to find that relatives or friends do not understand the importance of diet and may even criticize them for not serving meats or other less-than-healthy foods to their children.

Old beliefs die hard, so it's not surprising that many people cling to outdated ideas, particularly if they haven't read about the scientific reports that support a plant-based diet for children as well as adults. The results of some of these studies form the basis of this book; they represent the most current information we have about nutrition. It is now clear that meals built from vegetables, grains, fruits, and legumes make up the most nutritious possible diet.

You can certainly quote these studies and try to reassure anxious

Eating Away from Home

Feeding children a nutritious diet is worry-free when they are young and take all their meals at home. Mom and Dad prepare breakfast, lunch, dinner, and between-meal snacks, and know exactly what goes on the plate and into the mouth. It's a different story when our kids go to preschool, play dates, and parties.

I remember the conflict I felt when the oldest of my three children was asked to a birthday party. She was a cheerful, energetic four-year-old at the time and was giddy with excitement over her first real invitation. Her mother, on the other hand, was a bit worried. My daughter had never tasted dairy-based ice cream, and the occasional cake I baked was milk- and egg-free. I didn't want her to begin a lifetime of poor eating habits, but neither did I want to cast a shadow over the party by warning her away from the fat-laden sweets. In the end I said nothing and hoped for the best.

As it turned out, I needn't have worried. The children were so busy tearing around the room after balloons they hardly noticed the heaping plates of ice cream and cake set out on the table. My daughter did taste the dessert, but put her fork down after one bite. She didn't like the way it felt on her tongue, she told me later; except for that, she happily related, it was a great party.

I have found that my children do not miss fatty foods from animal sources because they never ate them at home. Nor do they feel awkward or different at social events, as they have learned to say, politely and simply, "No, thank you." They look for, and fill up on, the healthy foods they have learned to like at home.

KATHY GUILLERMO

relatives. You might try handing them a copy of this book. But the best answer to their questions will be the good health of your children. Babies and toddlers who grow up with healthy diets are less likely to suffer from food allergies, colic, indigestion, overweight, ear infections, and other common childhood illnesses. Regular visits to the pediatrician should reassure everyone that your baby or toddler is just as healthy—indeed, healthier—than children raised on the unhealthy foods that are all too common today.

One day your children will thank you. They will understand the health advantage you have given them, and they will be grateful.

7

Growing Kids

During the toddler years, children experiment with tastes and textures. They learn how to handle food and get most of it, at least, into their mouths, and they begin to form strong opinions about food. As they start into grade school, their food choices will broaden, and they will be naturally curious about cooking and where their food comes from. You can put that curiosity to good use by including them in the process of purchasing, preparing, and serving food. When children are involved in these activities, they are much more likely to try new foods and develop new tastes.

In a fascinating study done in third- and fifth-grade classrooms, Cornell University researchers taught students about the culture and history of different cuisines and actually had them prepare a few simple foods in the classroom. They learned where grains, beans, greens, or other healthy foods come from, and how they are transformed into nourishing meals. Students kept notebooks about the foods, wrote down recipes, and even created some of their own, using the ingredients they had learned about. When they were later offered these foods as part of the lunchroom fare, they ate ten times more of them than students from classrooms who had not received these interactive nutrition lessons. The children who had learned how to cook these new foods were happily eating all different kinds of greens such as collards and kale, hot peppers, capers, beans of all types, vegetable sushi, Chinese dumplings, and a variety of other healthy foods and dishes. Many took their new knowledge home to their parents, giving them a chance to try new, healthy foods.

From this study the researchers developed a curriculum called Food Is Elementary, which has been successfully used in many U.S. schools. It asks students to smell, taste, cook with, and appreciate the aesthetics of the food they are learning about, engaging all their senses. The teachers work with the students to develop a real sense of taste by having the children put the food in their mouths and noticing it while they count to three. When they spend a few seconds to identify flavor differences, the students come to prefer fresh, healthy plant foods.

You can use similar techniques with your children at home by inviting them to help you make the family meal. Even very young children can safely wash vegetables, tear lettuce, stir batter, roll out dough, and so forth. As your child's dexterity improves, teach him or her all the steps to make one or more favorite dishes such as a salad, bean burrito, or fruit smoothie. Many children delight in mastering a recipe or two. You might encourage them to write them down in a notebook.

If it takes more time than you can spare to include your small children in regular meal preparations, you may want to have special cook-together times—for example, on occasional Sunday afternoons. You could use this time to make a large casserole or soup that can be used throughout the week or frozen for later use.

One fun activity is to make a basic dish that your child enjoys, such as oatmeal, and gather a few ingredients you can mix in, such as fruits, nuts, or spices. Then, together make very small batches of different flavor combinations. Taste each one, rank them from favorite to least favorite, and compare your preferences. Cooking together with a small child will not only help him or her to build useful skill, but also may offer you some insights into your child's preferences and creativity.

Building Creativity in the Kitchen

Mom invited my brother and me to join her in the kitchen when we were very little—cooking was something fun that we did together. Over the years she showed us a whole lot of kitchen skills—like how to bake a perfect fruit pie (make double the amount of dough you need so it won't matter if some is snitched, and use half again as much filling as the recipe calls for); how to adapt a recipe; how to chop, dice, mince, slice, and pare; and how to tell when green beans are cooked to perfection. Then came lessons on basics of meal planning—every plate should be colorful and have a grain or a potato, a main dish, and at least one and preferably two vegetables.

Then she cut me loose in the kitchen. When I came home after school she would say something like "There are mushrooms and tofu in the fridge. And I got some really nice spinach at the market today. Why don't you do something with them this evening?" She kept a stocked freezer and pantry. I didn't shop or plan ahead. I'd just see what was in the kitchen and turn it into dinner. Through this experience I learned that creating healthy meals is challenging, enjoyable, and rewarding.

AMY JOY LANOU, PH.D.

These are the years when children learn, or don't learn, to enjoy a wide variety of food and when they learn to experiment with new foods and flavors. These are very important lessons for the rest of life.

Balanced Nutrition for Grade School Children

Meal planning for kindergarten through sixth graders is similar to that for toddlers except that your older child will need more food from each of the New Four Food Groups, as shown in the following table.

DAILY MEAL PLANNING FOR GRADE SCHOOL CHILDREN

5–6-YEAR-OLDS	7–12-YEAR-OLDS	DESCRIPTIONS
Whole grains, breads, cereals: 6 servings	Whole grains, breads, cereals: 7 servings	Serving: 1 slice bread, $\frac{1}{2}$ bun or bagel, $\frac{1}{2}$ cup cooked cereal, grain, or pasta, $\frac{3}{4}$ to 1 cup ready-to-eat cereal, crackers. Choose whole grains whenever possible.
Vegetables: $\frac{1}{4}$ cup dark green vegetables; $\frac{1}{4}$ to $\frac{1}{2}$ cup other vegetables	Vegetables: 1 serving dark green vegetables; 3 servings other vegetables	Dark green vegetables: broccoli, kale, collard greens, mustard greens, and bok choy are good choices. Other vegetables: any and all, fresh or frozen, raw or cooked. Serving: $\frac{1}{2}$ cup cooked or 1 cup raw
Legumes, nuts, seeds, milks: $\frac{1}{2}$ to 1 cup legumes; 3 servings soy milk or other nondairy milk	Legumes, nuts, seeds, milks: 2 servings legumes; 3 servings soy milk or other nondairy milk	Legumes: beans, peas, tofu, and lentils cooked until soft. Serving nondairy milk: 1 cup. Serving legumes: $\frac{1}{2}$ cup cooked beans, tofu, or peas. Nuts and seeds: optional in small amounts (1–2 tbsp).

5–6- YEAR-OLDS	7–12- YEAR-OLDS	DESCRIPTIONS
Fruits: 1 to 2 cups	Fruits: 3 servings	Fruits: any and all, fresh or frozen, raw or cooked.
		Serving: 1 medium fruit, ½ cup fruit chunks, ¼ cup dried fruit, ¾ cup fruit juice

Adapted from Virginia Messina and Mark Messina, *The Dietitian's Guide to Vegetarian Diets*. (Gaithersburg, Md.: Aspen, 1996).

You are doing your children a big favor by building their meals from vegetables, grains, legumes, and fruits. They will have an easier time staying slim, and will most likely avoid a whole host of childhood health problems, from acne and constipation to asthma and Type 1 diabetes. And they will be way ahead of many of their peers in terms of avoiding serious illnesses later in life.

The American Academy of Pediatrics recommends a diet for children that is moderately low in fat (30% of calories), low in saturated fat (<10% of calories), and low in cholesterol (<300mg/day). Nonetheless, according to a major national survey, most children in the United States aren't hitting these goals. The average child consumes too much total fat (36% of calories) and way too much saturated fat (13% of calories). And, shocking as it may sound, a Centers for Disease Control and Prevention report on obesity in America found that 60 percent of overweight five-to ten-year-olds already have at least one risk factor for heart disease, such as raised blood pressure or insulin levels.

A study of eight-to ten-year-olds with moderately elevated cholesterol levels showed that a low-fat diet modestly reduced cholesterol and provided adequate nutrition to maintain growth, iron stores, and psychological well-being. Many more positive health results are likely when children follow healthy, vegan eating habits right from the start and maintain this low-fat, vitamin- and fiber-rich, cholesterol-free eating style throughout their lives. Happily, many pediatricians who understand the importance of diet for children's health now recommend using the New Four Food Groups to meet kids' nutritional needs and help them avoid animal fat and cholesterol. Of course, it is not a "diet" at all—just a very different way of eating than most of us grew up with.

Grade school students may eat many of their meals away from the home, and this presents new challenges. During this time your children will likely realize that many of their friends do not eat quite so healthfully as your family does. While you may serve veggieburgers or veggie hot dogs, many friends will still eat the original, high-fat varieties. It is important to talk to your kids about why your family eats as it does, encouraging them to value these healthy practices.

Healthy Snacking Habits

Busy families sometimes have trouble fitting in three healthy meals each day. Like it or not, snacking has become an important contributor to daily food intake. According to a U.S. Department of Agriculture (USDA) survey of nearly ten thousand children, twice as many kids today eat snack foods such as crackers, popcorn, pretzels, and corn chips as did kids just twenty years ago. Soda consumption has increased 37 percent for six-to-nine-year-olds during the same time period. While children are eating extra calories, many still fall short of meeting their needs for vitamins and minerals such as vitamin E, vitamin B_6, zinc, and iron.

What this means is that extra care needs to be taken to make certain your child's snacks are every bit as healthful as the meals you serve. To do this, use the same guidelines for snack planning as for meal planning. Many healthy convenient options can be found within each of the New Four Food Groups.

A Parents' Idea List for Healthy Snacks

Baby carrots and other plain cut veggies

Breadsticks or pita chips with hummus

Fresh fruits

Dried fruits, especially raisins

Nuts, especially mixed with dried fruit

Cheerios or other cereal in a bag

Toast with fruit spread or nut butters

Soy ice cream

Almond butter and jelly sandwiches

Frozen bananas blended with a little nondairy milk

Chunks of plain avocados

Raw mushrooms

Applesauce or other fruit cups

Apple slices with hazelnut butter

Source: From a parents' discussion group on www.vegsource.com 2000.

Choosing Whole Foods

Selecting unprocessed foods such as whole grains or fresh fruits and vegetables more often and highly processed foods less often makes getting the right amount of nutrients much easier. Far more health benefit is obtained from eating, for example, a juicy, raw tomato slice than an equal amount of the much more highly processed ketchup.

Processing certainly offers some benefits by increasing our ability to store fresh produce for later use (such as in canning and freezing), retarding spoilage (refrigeration and salting), and improving convenience (frozen meals or microwaveable dinners). However, food processing also has brought some new problems.

Food that has undergone multiple processing steps nearly always loses some of its important nutrients and often picks up substances we generally can do without. For example, take the transformation of a potato into a potato chip. First, its nutrient-rich peel is discarded, thus losing much of its fiber, iron, and calcium. Then it is sliced, washed, and fried—adding fat, removing water, and destroying B vitamins. Next it is salted and sometimes flavored with spices and colored with artificial colorings. Finally, chemical preservatives are added to make the chips last longer on the shelf. The resulting product, a serving of potato chips, has crunch and convenience but has seventy times as much fat, twenty times as much salt, half the carbohydrates, and less than a third the amount of fiber and iron, vitamin C, and thiamin of a baked potato.

One widespread type of processing, called partitioning, causes particular problems with dietary balance. Partitioning occurs when some part of a food is separated from the rest. Examples include sugar taken from beets, oil extracted from peanuts or soybeans, and refined flour taken from whole grains. Nearly 70 percent of the U.S. food supply consists of partitioned foods that are almost completely devoid of fiber, vitamins, and minerals, including purified sugars, fats, and oils; refined flour; other milled grains; and alcohol. Less than a century ago our diet was made up almost entirely of whole foods. To have a healthy and nutritionally sound diet, no more than 20 percent of your family's daily fare—less is better—should come from these partitioned, highly processed foods. It's not as difficult as it sounds. You'll just need to be on the lookout for sugar, white flour, and fried foods.

Children often are the targets of companies marketing highly processed foods such as punches, cereals, candy, soda, and snacks. Teach them to be smart consumers by pointing out the difference between the food images they see on TV or in magazine ads and the actual food products. For example, punches and other beverages are sold with colorful images of fruit but often contain little or no fruit. Help them to be able to identify and seek out fresh, healthy, *whole* foods.

"Where Does My Food Come From?"

A good way to answer is to involve kids in the food production process itself. Children of all ages delight in going berry or apple picking, helping out in a garden, and visiting farms, farmers' markets, and even food processing plants or restaurants. Even a simple activity such as starting a windowsill garden or sprouting seeds in a jar offers some understanding of where foods come from.

You might let your children taste firsthand the difference between produce picked right from the garden and produce that has traveled many miles and waited weeks before making it to your table. Add to that an understanding of where meat, eggs, and milk come from by visiting farms where animals are being raised for this purpose, and children have a much easier time declining poor food choices.

Another useful activity is to trace the ingredients of a highly processed food from their source to the package. What whole foods were used to make each ingredient? What had to happen to turn them into ingredients? What is the difference in health value between the resultant processed food and the original whole foods? What happens to the parts of the whole foods that were not used?

Or try a simple exercise: Compare the number of ingredients on a popular brand of Spanish rice or similar food with a health food brand. The difference can be a real eye-opener.

Building Responsible Health Choices

Grade school children have lots of opportunities to make decisions about what foods they eat. They will likely be eating in other family members' homes; with their friends at parties or sleepovers; and, of course, at school.

In some of these instances you can smooth your child's way by letting other family members or parents know what kinds of foods you serve at home and by sending a dish-to-share to parties and overnights. Other parents usually appreciate learning about the food habits of their guests, and will be as accommodating as they can be.

Nonetheless, there will be times when your son or daughter will have to make some choices. You can prepare your child to make healthful decisions by talking about the advantages and disadvantages of different types of foods ahead of time, and teaching your child how to politely ask for foods or decline others. These skills will have lifelong value. You could even make a game out of going to fast-food restaurants and finding the most healthy items on the menus.

By showing your children a good example, offering them healthy foods so that they develop a taste for them, educating them about food and cooking, and allowing them to make choices, you will help them build a set of skills that will serve them well as they grow.

8

The Teen Years

They are the best of times and the worst of times. During the teen years children try new experiences, make their own decisions, and find rebellious ways to express themselves. Parents envy their boundless energy and recoil at their fashion sense. And you will find your role changing from a more direct one as teacher and guardian to a more supportive one as your child forges his or her own path. You can still offer your guidance, respect, and wisdom, and help your children learn from their experiences. And don't underestimate your importance as a role model for your teen's eating habits.

But the undeniable fact is, as children reach the teen years, their eating habits often take a turn for the worse. A study, published in 2000, observed the eating habits of students in the third grade and again in the eighth grade and found that, as teens, these students ate 41 percent less fruit and 25 percent fewer vegetables than they had as third graders. In eighth grade the students also drank much more soda and ate breakfast less often.

Many teens do not eat anywhere near five servings of fruits and vegetables a day. A nationwide survey found that only 15 percent of high school students met the five-a-day recommendations, while more than half did not eat any cooked vegetables. More than a third had no fruit on the day preceding the survey. In another study, from 1995, 30 to 40 percent of students had fruits and vegetables *less than once a day*. Overall the diets of teenagers are much like those of their parents—too high in fat and sugar, and low in fiber and complex carbohydrates.

On a more optimistic note, vegetarian diets are on the rise among teenagers. Adolescents tend to be drawn to meatless diets for environmental or animal rights reasons, and they stand to benefit healthwise from this choice. A study of the nutritional quality of adolescent vegetarian diets found that teen female vegetarians consumed 40 percent more fiber and 20 percent more vitamin C than their omnivorous peers. And, of course, animal fat and cholesterol are much less likely to make an appearance on their plates.

Meal Planning Guidelines
for Adolescents

The teen years are famous for rapid growth, big appetites, and the hormonal shifts associated with puberty. A child's fastest growth after infancy happens in the adolescent growth spurt, which typically lasts 1½ to 2 years and can occur anytime between ages 10 and 15. Nutrient and energy needs are especially high during this period, about 50 percent higher than adults on a body weight basis—and fluctuate throughout adolescence. Appetite generally follows growth, so you needn't worry whether your teens will eat enough food.

While parents are often concerned about the protein intake of vegetarian teens, this is one nutrient that they are almost never lacking. Because of the increased need for energy during these years, protein intake need only be about 7 to 8 percent of calories (45 to 59 grams/day). This is a smaller percentage of calories as protein than is recommended for adults (10 to 15%) and is less than the 10 to 12 percent of calories that vegans typically consume. What this means is that even if your teenager does no meal planning at all, but

Family Meals

At our house, dinnertime was always family time. While other families were busy with work, friends, school, sports, or whatever, our family of five had unusual success at making dinnertime a magnet—a real highlight of the day. In retrospect I have been trying to figure out what we did.

I'd like to say that we insisted on dinner at six o'clock with everybody there. But it was several years into the high school experience that I realized dinnertime was going pretty well without much insisting from me. Basically the kids really wanted to be there. The priority was to have everybody there, so we often moved dinnertime around to accommodate work and sports. Part of the reason was because my wife made great food, and every night seemed to be somebody's favorite meal. But the big draw was just the sheer fun of eating and talking together. Everyone eventually got a turn to tell what happened to them that day, victories, embarrassments, and all. It was the culmination of our days as we talked about everything; the news, sex, sports stories, friends, church, work, and weird neighbors. Dinnertime was a time for hearing and being heard. It also was a time for some richly sardonic ridicule and even an occasional food fight.

Now that the kids are grown and out of the house, I tend to look back on those times through the smoked glass of fond memories. I am still amazed that our kids really wanted to eat dinner together, and we all gladly made the sacrifices needed to have our time together.

MARTIN ROOT, PH.D.

does eat a variety of foods made from grains, beans, and vegetables, there is no need to worry about protein.

Teens have increased requirements for calcium, iron, zinc, and vitamin B_{12}. Appealing calcium sources for teenagers include fortified orange juice and all of the other calcium-fortified juices now appearing on the market; calcium-set tofu; almond butter; tahini; calcium-fortified soy or rice milk; textured vegetable protein used in chili, tacos, or "sloppy joes"; English muffins; and corn tortillas. Beans, figs, kale, collards, and mustard greens also are good sources.

Iron is especially important for adolescent girls, as their needs are higher than boys'. However, vegan teens actually have an easier time meeting their needs for iron, because strict vegetarian diets tend to be richer in iron than omnivorous ones. Also, because both calcium and cow's milk are inhibitors of iron absorption, the avoidance of dairy products by vegans helps, too.

Vegan teens need to supplement their diet with vitamin B_{12} or regularly consume B_{12}-fortified foods. As we saw in chapter 1, that is easy to do. Zinc, which is needed for many functions, including sexual maturation and growth, is available to teenagers in whole grains, nuts, and legumes.

Teens, like younger children, can meet these nutrient needs by simply building their meals using the New Four Food Groups and adding a standard multivitamin or any other good source of vitamin B_{12}. Daily meal planning guidelines are shown in the following table. Please note that the numbers of servings children need vary tremendously, depending on their size and activity levels. Some teens will need more, and others will need less at some times during these years.

Diet and Puberty

Scientists have known for a long time that nutrition affects how fast children grow, how soon their "growth spurt" arrives, and even the age of menarche, when a young woman first menstruates. Malnutrition due to food scarcity, severe dieting, or very high activity levels could all delay puberty or menarche. So, in the not-so-distant past, doctors and nutritionists thought that faster growth and an earlier age of menarche were signs of good health. Now we are coming to realize that bigger, faster, or sooner are not always better.

More gradual development may well be healthier overall. Physicians are especially concerned about the early ages at which children are reaching puberty, because girls who start their periods earlier have a higher risk of breast cancer later. In fact, one of the

DAILY MEAL PLANNING GUIDELINES
FOR ADOLESCENTS

Whole grains, breads, cereals: 10 servings

Serving: 1 slice bread, ½ bun or bagel, ½ cup cooked cereal, grain, or pasta, ¾ to 1 cup ready-to-eat cereal

Choose whole grains whenever possible.

Vegetables: 1–2 servings dark green vegetables; 3 servings other vegetables

Dark green vegetables: broccoli, kale, collard greens, mustard greens, and bok choy are good choices.

Other vegetables: any and all, fresh or frozen, raw or cooked.

Serving: ½ cup cooked or 1 cup raw

Legumes, nuts, seeds, milk: 3 servings legumes; 3 servings soy milk or other nondairy milk

Legumes: beans, peas, tofu, and lentils, veggieburgers, tempeh, etc.

Serving nondairy milk: 1 cup.

Serving legumes: ½ cup cooked beans, tofu, or peas.

Nuts and seeds: optional in small amounts (1–4 tbsp).

Fruits: 4 servings

Fruits: any and all, fresh or frozen, raw or cooked.

Serving: 1 medium fruit, ½ cup fruit chunks, ¼ cup dried fruit, ¾ cup fruit juice.

Adapted from Virginia Messina and Mark Messina, *The Dietitian's Guide to Vegetarian Diets,* (Gaithersburg, Md.: Aspen, 1996).

parts of the Western diet that is thought to affect the age of menarche, dairy products, raises levels of a factor in the blood called *insulinlike growth factor I* levels. Higher IGF-I levels are linked to increased risks of breast, ovarian, and prostate cancer.

Here is the problem: Kids grow up on a diet that is rich in meat, dairy, and high-fat convenience foods and therefore high in fat, animal protein, and calories. This dietary pattern, along with the low consumption of fruits and vegetables mentioned earlier, is thought to be responsible, at least in part, for the growth of excess body fat and higher body weights of today's teenagers. And evidence suggests that these dietary practices also may be responsible for women passing through puberty at younger and younger ages. A recent study from Harvard School of Public Health showed that girls who consumed more animal protein, rather than vegetable protein, went through menarche earlier. More calories, more meat, and more dairy products—these were all linked with premature growth and earlier menarche, even when these researchers controlled for body size. These foods distort the normal growth patterns and hormone balance of the body, and children show the effects all too clearly.

Studies in different parts of the world strongly support this connection. In Europe and North America, where meat is a dietary staple, sexual maturation occurs much earlier than in parts of Asia and Latin America where dietary staples come from plants—rice, vegetables, beans, or tortillas, for example—with much less use of animal products. Sadly, the gradual Westernization of Japan's diet after World War II was followed by a 2½-year drop in the average age of menarche in girls there.

Once your teen daughters have begun menstruating, they may be interested to learn that what they eat can reduce the pain of menstrual cramps. A recent study demonstrated that when women who suffer from menstrual pain shift to an entirely plant-based diet, with no added fat, most experience much less pain. This effect is thought to be due to reduced estrogen production and better estrogen excretion. It does not take long to see if the diet helps. Its benefits are usually felt in the first month.

Setting the Stage for Good Adult Health

The dietary pattern that is connected with early menarche—a diet including meat, dairy, and fat, while low in fruits, vegetables, and grains—is a major risk factor for many other problems, including heart disease, diabetes, obesity, and a surprising number of cancers. Adolescents who, instead, consume a health-promoting diet built from the New Four Food Groups set the stage for good adult health.

Two recent studies illustrate this point. Scientists found that in blood tests, women who had higher levels of isoflavones, a compound found in a variety of plants, especially soybeans, had a 50 percent lower risk of breast cancer. And in a study of African American and Hispanic teens, blood pressure was lower in teens who consumed the greatest amount of folate, a B vitamin found in many fruits, vegetables, and grains. And vegetarian adults have significantly lower blood pressure than their omnivorous peers.

Overall, a healthier diet means a healthier body. In general, vegan teens find they have slimmer bodies and fewer health problems than their meat-eating friends.

Helping Your Child Stick with It

The ease with which vegetarians stick with this healthy dietary pattern is influenced by a variety of factors. If your children have convictions about the welfare of animals or reducing impact on the environment, or have a clear understanding of the health value of good eating habits, they will be more likely to maintain this diet throughout their lives. Having the shopping, dining out, and cooking skills in place will make it easier for them to continue eating healthfully when they move out of the house and are fully responsible for getting their own meals.

And family support is key, both while your kids are under your roof and long after they leave. When family members join in healthy eating habits, avoid tempting a child with unhealthy foods, and support older kids with healthy cookbooks or other appropriate gifts, they do a world of good.

If a Family Member Doesn't Understand

My grandfather was a family farmer who lived in a rural area in Pennsylvania. When I told him as a teenager that I had decided to be a vegetarian, he was appalled. He told me in complete sincerity and with concern that I would die if I did not eat meat. At that time I tried to explain to him that I had learned from my schooling and outside reading that vegetarian diets were better for the planet and were every bit as healthy as the diet he grew up on, if not more so. He remained unconvinced, but honored my stubbornness and choice by not talking to me about it again. Luckily, my parents were supportive of my decision, and he lived long enough to see me grow into a healthy adult.

AMY JOY LANOU, PH.D.

The New Four Food Groups offer the same benefits to adolescents as they do to people of all ages. By encouraging your teenagers to experiment with new foods from plant sources, try new recipes, and taste cuisines from around the world, they'll mature into a lifetime of healthy eating.

PART III

Lifelong Health

9

Foods and Common Health Problems

The foods children eat not only affect their health in the seemingly distant future—the risk of heart attacks, chronic weight problems, cancer, diabetes, etc.—but also what children eat can affect their health right now. Many childhood ailments, including allergies, asthma, ear infections, constipation, juvenile-onset Type 1 diabetes, skin conditions, and many other problems, have direct links to diet.

Fighting Infections

Among the most critical functions in a child's body—or your own, for that matter—is the immune system's vital job of fighting off infections that find their way into your body. It also has to spot abnormal cells such as cancer cells, and eliminate them before they can cause harm. The immune system uses potent weapons to help you and your children stay well, and it does a remarkably good job when you consider that bacteria, viruses, and various misfit cells turn up in our bodies every day. Foods can power up the immune system or, if they are the wrong choices, weaken it and leave the body vulnerable to invaders.

The immune system is actually a team, with different cells serving different functions. Key players are B cells, T cells, and natural killer cells. B cells make antibodies, protein molecules that attach to the surface of bacteria or other foreign cells and attract other white blood cells to come to destroy the undesirables. T cells swallow invaders whole. Some T cells direct the traffic of the immune system, telling the B cells when to stop and start making antibodies. And, just as with most good leaders, they will join in the battles as well. Natural killer cells search for foreign abnormal or infected cells and destroy them. Other immune system cells (basophils and mast cells) release histamine that causes cells to break open, allowing other scavenger cells to clean up the mess.

This team is quick and efficient, and without it you could not survive. Even so, it functions a bit awkwardly sometimes. In fact, much of the discomfort associated with the flu or a cold has to do with the actions the immune system takes in the effort to destroy the invading organism, rather than the actions of the organisms themselves. Nonetheless, you want to take very good care of your immune system.

Like many parents, you may already realize that the foods your children eat can make a difference to the immune strength. Many families drink extra orange juice or eat extra fruit when someone in the household feels a cold coming on, or will offer hot soup or hot tea to a child with a sore throat. The vitamin C in fruit juice bolsters your immunity, as do beta-carotene and vitamin E. And warm liquids increase blood circulation to your child's sore throat, bringing in the army of immune system defenders.

Building these nutrients into your family's daily routine is easy. Brightly colored fruits and vegetables are the best sources of vitamin C and beta-carotene. Vitamin E is found in vegetables, grains, nuts, and seeds. A diet rich in these foods will help keep your immune system strong and ready to fight off infection as effectively as possible. Vitamin C has been shown both to reduce the likelihood that a cold will arrive and to shorten its course if it should catch you.

Your immune system's success in its search-and-destroy

Too Much of a Good Thing?

When I was teaching about problems of overusing vitamins in a college nutrition class, one student told this story. When he was younger, he was a sickly child who often had stomachaches and chronically had problems with diarrhea. His parents were very attentive to his health and had tried many ways to help him. Sadly, it wasn't until he was about ten years old that a doctor learned that they had been giving him large daily doses of vitamin C since he was a small child (500 to 1000 mg), presumably, to keep him well. The recommended amount for nine-to-thirteen-year-olds is only 45 mg/day, the amount in a half cup of strawberries or 4 ounces of orange juice. When the doctor suggested that he stop taking the vitamin C pills, his stomachaches and diarrhea cleared up almost overnight.

There are certainly important roles for supplements, but his story illustrates why most pediatricians and nutritionists recommend that you and your children get immune-boosting nutrients from foods instead. And don't worry if you eat a little more of the vitamins you need in food—your body seems to be able to handle the extra better when they come in the original package.

AMY JOY LANOU, PH.D.

missions is also influenced by the amount of fat and cholesterol in the diet. Too much cholesterol in the bloodstream interferes with the white blood cells' ability to work. In turn, your cholesterol level is influenced by how much saturated fat and cholesterol you eat. As you know by now, avoiding food from animal sources—that means meats (all kinds), eggs, and dairy products—goes a long way toward keeping your blood cholesterol levels low. Fruits, vegetables, grains, and legumes are always cholesterol-free and usually are very low in saturated fat.

Keeping your fat intake low is important. White blood cells can't function in an oil slick. This is true for all types of fat. Fryer grease, salad dressings, and added oils can really slow down white blood cells, just as animal fats can. An immune-boosting menu, then, is one that avoids foods from animal sources and keeps vegetable fats to a minimum.

In addition to providing your child with healthy low-fat vegetarian foods, you'll also want to avoid the spread of infection. The main way colds and flu are spread is via physical contact. So teaching your children to wash their hands frequently and thoroughly and to avoid putting their fingers in their noses and mouths will help them avoid picking up germs.

Allergies

Approximately fifty million people in the United States sneeze throughout the fall, itch when they eat peanuts, wheeze when they pet cats, or show other symptoms of allergy. Some are even at risk of dying from severe allergic reactions to various substances that are benign or only slightly irritating to most people. And when allergy symptoms—hives, sneezing, runny nose, migraine—are not life-threatening, they can certainly affect your child's ability to get the most out of life.

Experts disagree on the precise definition of "allergy." Some call any sensitivity reaction an allergy, while others hold that only reactions involving a specific antibody called IgE are true allergies. No matter how you define them, the basic events happening in the body and the strategies for coping with them are similar.

In essence, an allergic reaction is one that mobilizes the immune system inappropriately. Like a case of mistaken identity, the immune system reacts to a harmless substance as though it were an invading bacteria or virus. It mobilizes antibodies that attach themselves to the allergen and to white blood cells packed with histamine. The combination is explosive: The cells break open, spewing histamine into the tissues, causing swelling, itching, and other familiar symptoms of allergy. Scavenger cells eventually arrive to remove the debris, but in the meantime you'll feel pretty miserable. Symptoms can appear virtually anywhere in the body, but commonly in the skin, lining of the gut, lungs, sinuses, or head.

The tendency to have allergies is partly genetic. If one parent suffers from allergies, a child has a 30 percent chance of also developing allergic symptoms. If both parents have allergies, the risk climbs to about 65 percent. Whether or not the genetic tendency lives itself out or not depends on many factors, little understood at this time. Nonetheless, if your child is allergy-prone, there are certain things you can do to lessen the symptoms. For example, to reduce the sneezes and itchy eyes of hay fever at night, keep bedroom windows closed if possible. Units that filter the air are readily available; look for one containing a HEPA filter, excellent for removing allergens of all types. For allergies to animals, dust, and molds, it helps to keep a very clean house, wash hands and face after contact with animals, and wash or replace bed pillows frequently.

Foods also can influence allergies or sensitivities. For example, quercetin, a natural phytochemical in many vegetables, dampens allergic responses by inhibiting the release of histamine. You'll find it in red grapes, yellow squash, shallots and broccoli. Onions also contain large amounts of quercetin along with other compounds.

Vitamin C also works to dampen inflammatory responses in the body. And plant foods, generally, seem to reduce allergies, compared to diets loaded with meats and dairy products. A British study found that children from India eating their traditional diet had far fewer allergic symptoms than their schoolmates eating a typical Western diet. The Indian diet was richer in vegetables and contained less meat and fewer packaged and processed foods than the traditional British diet.

Food Allergies

Many people suffer from allergies or sensitivities to foods, commonly milk, wheat, peanuts, and soy, although almost any food can trigger symptoms in certain people. Just as with other allergies, food allergies involve an overreactivity of the immune system. For various reasons, antibodies that are designed to protect us from disease react against certain proteins in foods, causing bloating, headaches, hives, and diarrhea.

Unlike inhaled allergens such as ragweed or dust, food allergens enter the body through the intestinal tract. For food allergies, one special type of antibody, called IgA, plays a particularly important role. Your digestive tract is ordinarily lined with IgA, which helps attack food allergens before they can inappropriately "leak" across the lining of the intestine and cause trouble. Children with food sensitivities often have unusually low levels of IgA in their blood, and certain foods can aggravate the problem. Foods containing hydrogenated oils, such as margarine, appear to encourage this destructive permeability of the intestine. The problem is their trans-fatty acids, which are formed as the manufacturer hardens a liquid oil, such as soybean or corn oil, into a solid fat that you can slice or spread.

Stress also can decrease the amount of IgA in your body. This may help explain why food allergies are often worse during high-stress periods. Whether your child's symptoms are caused by a true food allergy or by food sensitivities of other kinds, avoiding the foods that trigger them can help. Start by building a diet from the New Four Food Groups and avoiding those foods that are known to cause your child's undesirable reactions. If the allergies do not clear up, try avoiding other foods that are known to cause allergies in other individuals. Dairy products are a surprisingly common contributor to sensitivities of all kinds, as we'll see in more detail shortly. The problem is the milk *protein,* not the fat, so skim products are of no help. Try rice milk or soy milk instead. Eggs are common allergens, as are peanuts and other nuts, fish, corn, or wheat.

Once you track down which foods trigger the reactions, a dietary plan known as the "rotation diet" can be helpful. This diet does not prescribe or forbid any particular food; rather, it suggests that children avoid eating the same foods every day. The idea is that the body can become oversensitized to certain food components if it has to deal with them constantly, whereas if it is in contact with them only infrequently—not more often than every four days—it is less likely to develop a sensitivity or an allergy to them.

Try to vary your foods from day to day, particularly foods that are common allergens, such as soy, wheat, citrus, or potatoes. For example, if your child tends to have food allergies, it's probably wise to rotate his or her morning orange juice with apple and other juices and fruits. And try substituting corn bread or rice crackers for wheat toast.

The rotation diet is certainly helpful in avoiding the development of new food sensitivities. With already existing sensitivities, if they are not severe, you could try eating a small portion of the offending food once every four or five days or so. Some people can avoid triggering reactions this way, while others will have to completely remove allergy-provoking foods from their diets. Experiment cautiously with your child's diet to see what works best. Foods such as dairy products or eggs that contribute to many different health problems are best left out of the diet altogether.

Cow's Milk Intolerance

Many people have trouble digesting milk. For most, the problem is lactose, the main sugar in milk. It requires the enzyme lactase in order to be broken down into its simpler sugars, glucose and galactose. Virtually all infants have this enzyme, but as they grow older, most gradually lose these enzymes, along with the ability to digest this sugar. The lactose passes into the large intestine undigested and causes gas, cramps, bloating, and diarrhea, because it is broken down by the bacteria that normally live there.

People of northern European ancestry are often still able to digest lactose on into their adult years, but 70 percent of African Americans, 90 percent of Asian Americans, 53 percent of Mexican Americans, and 74 percent of Native Americans lose this ability. In fact, anyone whose ancestry is African, Asian, Native American, Arab, Jewish, Hispanic, Italian, or Greek is likely to be less able to tolerate milk products as they become adults. This is not a disease. It is a totally normal state of affairs, found in 75 percent of people worldwide, and is simply a reminder that many adults are not well adapted to drinking cow's milk.

Chronic diarrhea is the most common symptom of cow's milk intolerance in children. However, recent reports published in the *New England Journal of Medicine* in 1998 have also linked chronic constipation to cow's milk intolerance. In one, 68 percent of children with chronic constipation got better when soy milk was given instead of cow's milk. Others researchers have confirmed that many children with chronic constipation get better when dairy products are removed from the diet.

While lactase enzyme pills are now available to assist lactose-intolerant individuals in digesting milk sugar, there is no need for your children to drink milk after they are weaned from breast milk and certainly no need for milk from another species. In fact, your child will avoid other possible health concerns by getting his or her nutrients from plant foods (see chapter 5). Because so many children have problems with dairy products, it is best not to introduce these foods into their diets at all.

Recurrent Ear Infections

Otitis media, or recurrent ear infections, is a major cause of acquired hearing loss in children and one of the most common reasons for visits to the pediatrician in the United States. While doctors still do not fully understand all the causes of this problem, in recent years food allergies, particularly cow's milk allergies, have emerged as a major contributor. In a study of eighty-one recurrent-ear-infection patients aged 1½ to 9 years with food sensitivities, elimination diets resolved the problem for 86 percent of the children. Cow's milk was the most common food allergy, with wheat, eggs, peanuts, and soy close behind. Another study concluded that children with cow's milk allergy in infancy have an elevated risk for recurrent ear infections throughout childhood. While we still have much to learn about the causes of ear infections, if your child has repeated problems with them, investigating potential food causes is well worthwhile, and avoiding the common triggers is a good place to start.

Asthma

Asthma is a repeated constriction of the bronchial tubes that results in wheezing and difficulty in breathing. Childhood asthma is a major concern of parents and physicians worldwide. It is often difficult to treat and, in severe cases, can be deadly. Many researchers in various parts of the world have observed a connection between the adoption of an affluent Westernized urban lifestyle and an increased risk of asthma and allergic disease. Possible factors include increasing pollution; parental smoking; and, of course, dietary changes.

In a study of fifty 1½-to-6-year-olds with asthma, when the children were challenged with milk and egg allergens, some had asthmatic or allergic reactions. Adults with asthma who switched to a vegan diet for a full year had marked improvements in their health. They needed less medication and had fewer and less severe attacks. Relief from allergies to dairy may be partially responsible for this improvement.

Another study linked asthma to low fruit and vegetable consumption, inadequate vitamin E, and higher numbers of visits to fast food restaurants. A diet rich in fresh fruit has been shown to have a positive effect on lung health, including reduced risk of asthma and of lung cancer. Along the same lines, adequate intake of foods rich in the antioxidant nutrients, beta-carotene, vitamin C, vitamin E, and selenium, reduces the risk of asthma.

Treatment of asthma has two parts: management of acute attacks as they happen, and preventing new attacks. The latter is very important, because the drugs used to deal with acute attacks are strong, some are addictive, and they tend to be suppressive rather than curative.

An asthma prevention diet is built from fruits, vegetables, beans, and grains, eliminates all dairy products, includes lots of clean water, and keeps vegetable oils (especially transfatty acids) to a minimum. If more improvement is needed, experiment with the elimination of wheat, corn, soy, and sugar to see if asthma improves.

Type 1 Diabetes

When children develop diabetes it is generally because they are not producing enough of the hormone insulin, which is responsible for helping the body move sugars and proteins from the bloodstream into the cells. Insulin is produced in the pancreas. In recent years, consumption of cow's milk during infancy and childhood has been implicated as part of the cause of this irreversible disease.

Here's how scientists think this happens: When small children consume dairy products, some of the proteins from the milk can pass through the gut into the bloodstream. If these proteins arrive in the bloodstream intact, the immune system fires up and makes antibodies to them. And this is when the trouble starts. These antibodies attack not only the milk proteins but also the insulin-producing cells in the pancreas, because they are similar in structure. Later, when the child gets a virus, antibody production is increased, and the pancreas comes under renewed attack. Eventually, in some children, so many of these cells are destroyed that the child can no longer make enough insulin to process the sugars and other carbohydrates the child eats. This child will be diagnosed with Type 1 diabetes and treated with regular insulin injections.

While this is likely only one of several ways that diabetes develops, the evidence supporting this connection between milk and diabetes is quite strong. In 1994, the American Academy of Pediatrics reviewed ninety studies addressing this question and concluded that cow's milk protein may indeed be an important factor in the development of diabetes and that avoiding cow's milk exposure may delay or prevent the disease in susceptible children. To reduce the risk of diabetes, mothers should breastfeed their children and strictly avoid giving them milk or other dairy products.

As we have seen, a surprising number of childhood ailments are connected directly or indirectly to food. A healthy diet, as described in chapters 1 through 8, will help your child build a strong immune system, and stay healthy and active in childhood and throughout life.

10

Feeding the Mind

A healthy diet is essential for the proper functioning of all body systems, including the brain's ability to perceive, think, and remember. There are countless theories about foods that affect a child's attention span, memory, and intelligence quotient. Many parents suspect, for example, that sugar causes hyperactivity and decreases a child's attention span. Other speculations declare chocolate, artificial colors, and preservatives as significantly affecting a child's cognitive development. The truth is that researchers and doctors are not entirely sure whether these speculations are correct.

Each child is unique in his or her own learning style, which makes it difficult to directly link differences in energy level and cognition to specific dietary or environmental factors. To further complicate things for parents, the media often jump on the "latest findings," leaving you confused and frustrated about what's good or bad for your children. A few things are certain, however. Breast-feeding improves IQ. Having a good breakfast helps learning. A plant-based diet, low in refined sugars throughout life, is what's best for overall health and possibly even the development of your child's brain. Concerns about artificial additives have turned out to be well founded for some kids but irrelevant for others. This chapter will provide details on these and other important issues.

Breastfeeding and Cognitive Development

Breastfeeding your child has a number of advantages, as we saw in chapter 4. In addition to these important health benefits, a number of studies have shown that breastfed children score higher on intelligence tests than children who were formula-fed. Better cognitive function can lead to higher grades in school; better job performance; greater income; and ease in interacting with classmates, friends, and relatives. A child's intellectual development is also influenced by a number of factors related to family or environment, such as smoking, parental intelligence and education, socioeconomic status, size of the family, birth order, and population density. But even after adjusting for these factors, breastfed infants still show a 3-point higher IQ on average, than those who were formula-fed. Breastfeeding makes an even bigger difference for premature and low-birth-weight infants, giving them an advantage of 5 IQ points, on average. It also has been suggested that breastfed children have fewer emotional or behavioral problems, and fewer neurological disturbances later in life. Some researchers attribute these benefits to the healthy combination of fats in human breast milk, which are quite different from those in cow's milk. However, cow's milk differs in many other respects as well, including the amount and type of protein it contains, and the levels of certain vitamins, among others. If breastfeeding your child is not possible, there are a number of soy-based infant formulas available that are nutrient-dense and that will promote your child's healthy growth and development.

Breakfast and Learning in Children

Starting your day with a healthy breakfast is a good idea, whether you're a child going to school or an adult headed for work. It prepares you for the active day that lies ahead. If you miss breakfast and your overnight fasting period is extended, your blood sugar level declines. This can trigger a stress response that disturbs alertness and memory. Breakfast also is an important component of our total daily nutrient requirements. Vitamin and mineral deficiencies alone can affect cognition and attention span.

The best evidence that breakfast improves intellect and memory has come in studies giving a morning meal to kids who had been undernourished. For them, breakfast makes a huge difference. Less certain are the effects of breakfast on the cognitive function of otherwise well-nourished children. Although no definitive conclusions have been reached, it is possible that the problem-solving performance of all children is improved by the consumption of breakfast.

Breakfast doesn't have to be an exhausting affair for you or your child. A bowl of cereal with soy milk and a glass of juice is the favorite of many youngsters. Having a variety of cereals on hand may add to the appeal of breakfast for your child. Other quick ideas include toaster waffles with raw fruit, whole grain toast with peanut butter and jelly, or oatmeal and raisins. If you're looking for extra protein, veggie sausages, tofu scramble, or even a small serving of chickpeas will meet your needs. Some people aren't hungry first thing in the morning. If this is the case with your child, don't force it. Instead, offer something small such as a glass of juice, soy milk, or rice milk and then pack a midmorning snack with a small sandwich, fruit, or a granola bar.

Nutrition for Hyperactivity and Attention Problems

Attention-deficit/hyperactivity disorder has gained a lot of attention in recent years. An "attention deficit" simply means having trouble staying focused on one thing for more than a few minutes. It often comes with hyperactivity. Parents and teachers often describe hyperactive children as restless, unable to sit still, incapable of finishing projects, fidgety, and talkative. Hyperactivity occurs in both sexes, but more commonly in boys than in girls.

Naturally, ADHD presents real challenges in the classroom setting. It's nearly impossible to learn when you can't sit still or can't focus your attention on one project for more than a few minutes. Many children are prescribed methylphenidate (Ritalin), or dextroamphetamine, to help them focus their attention and sit still in the classroom. Despite controversy surrounding the possible overuse

Signs of ADHD

A doctor will diagnose Attention-deficit/hyperactivity disorder if your child has had significant signs of inattention, hyperactivity, or both for at least six months.

Here are the signs of inattention (look for at least six of these):

1. often fails to give close attention to details or makes careless mistakes in schoolwork, work, or other activities
2. often has difficulty sustaining attention in tasks or play activities
3. often does not seem to listen when spoken to directly
4. often does not follow through on instructions and fails to finish schoolwork, chores, or duties in the workplace (not due to oppositional behavior or failure to understand instructions)
5. often has difficulty organizing tasks and activities
6. often avoids, dislikes, or is reluctant to engage in tasks that require sustained mental effort (such as schoolwork or homework)
7. often loses things necessary for tasks or activities (e.g., toys, school assignments, pencils, books, or tools)
8. is often easily distracted by extraneous stimuli
9. is often forgetful in daily activities

Here are the signs of hyperactivity (look for at least six of these):

1. often fidgets with hands or feet or squirms in seat
2. often leaves seat in classroom or in other situations in which remaining seated is expected
3. often runs about or climbs excessively in situations in which it is inappropriate (in adolescents or adults, may be limited to subjective feelings of restlessness)
4. often has difficulty playing or engaging in leisure activities quietly
5. is often "on the go" or often acts as if "driven by a motor"
6. often talks excessively
7. often blurts out answers before questions have been completed
8. often has difficulty awaiting turn

9. often interrupts or intrudes on others (e.g., butts into conver-
    sations or games)

Also, to make the diagnosis, some of these symptoms should
have started before age seven, the problem has to show up in at least
two settings (i.e., not only at school or only at home), and the condition has to interfere with the child's ability to function.

of these drugs, they clearly improve the attention span and behavior of some children and can be real life-savers. Far too many children are harmed by the failure to prescribe these drugs promptly,
due to the understandable reluctance of parents to use medications
for behavioral problems. It is important to recognize that attention
deficits often reflect subtle physical problems in the brain. So, for
many kids, all the counseling in the world is not as effective as sta-
bilizing medications.

There is also a role for diet, although it is still very much under
investigation. Sugar, food additives, chocolate, caffeine, mono-
sodium glutamate (MSG), and lead poisoning have all been considered possible triggers of attention deficit and hyperactivity. Most
experimental studies do not support the opinion that sugar intake
increases activity or promotes hyperactivity, and some have even
shown that activity levels decrease after sugar consumption. The
problem with the studies testing for behavior improvement with the
elimination of sugar is that many aspects of the diet change when
the sugar is taken out of the diet. For example, when refined sugars
such as candy and soft drinks are removed, these foods are typically
replaced with more nutrient-dense choices such as fruit and fruit
juice. So it may not necessarily be the removal of refined sugar
from the diet, but the addition of other necessary micronutrients
that improves the child's behavior and ability to learn.

Perhaps the most popular theory on diet and hyperactivity was
proposed Dr. Ben Feingold, who believed that removing synthetic
colors and flavors, as well as certain fruits and vegetables containing salicylates, from the diet could treat behavioral disturbances
in children. In Feingold's initial studies, about two-thirds of
hyperactive children improved with a diet change. It soon became
clear, however, that some children genuinely benefited from

the diet, while others got only a transient "placebo effect" that came from believing a diet change would help them. Just like the sugar studies, though, some hyperactive children do benefit from the elimination of food additives in their diet, while others do not.

Another researcher, Dr. Bonnie Kaplan, took the possible connection between diet and hyperactivity one step farther. In a study conducted in Alberta, Canada, in 1989, preschool-age boys with hyperactivity were given an experimental diet that eliminated not only artificial colors and flavors but also chocolate, mono-sodium glutamate, preservatives, caffeine, and any substance that families reported may affect their child's activity level. In addition, this diet was low in simple sugars such as candy and soft drinks, and free of dairy products if the family described cow's milk as a possible dietary problem. According to parents, more than half of the boys on the elimination diet showed a noteworthy improvement in behavior. Other improvements, including a reduction in bad breath and night awakenings, were reported for those on the exper-imental diet. The results of this study suggest that eliminating cer-tain foods from the diet of a child with hyperactivity may well be worth trying.

By feeding your child a healthy diet emphasizing whole grains, vegetables, legumes, and fruit, he or she is likely to avoid many of the hypothesized risk factors triggering attention deficit disorders. Also, recognizing food allergies or sensitivities and avoiding as many as you can will optimize your child's learning and development. Refer to chapter 1 for more detail on the New Four Food Groups and the numerous health benefits this eating plan holds for your child.

Your child with ADHD also may benefit from assigned tasks and a stable routine at home. When possible, engage your child in enjoyable projects that help him or her focus attention. Assign small, quickly finished tasks, and praise your child when the job is done. If your child is a willing participant, counseling and behavior modification may help, and parents often can benefit, too.

Autism

Autism is a complex developmental disability that usually appears before age three. It is not simply a psychological problem; it is also a neurological disorder that affects the functioning of the brain, disrupting social interactions and communication skills. According to the Centers for Disease Control and Prevention, autism is more prevalent in boys than in girls and occurs in as many as one in five hundred children.

Being characteristically self-absorbed makes it hard for affected kids to communicate with others and relate to the outside world. They may exhibit extreme withdrawal, even from their mother and father. In some cases, children become aggressive, self-injurious, or both. Children with autism thrive on sameness in people and things and can become quite attached to inanimate objects. They commonly demonstrate repeated body movements (hand flapping, rocking) and are resistant to change in routines. Few scientific studies show that food intake affects the behavior or cognitive function of a child with autism. However, it is possible that children with autism have either allergies to particular foods or difficulty digesting certain proteins in foods, and that, by eliminating these foods, behavioral symptoms will improve. Some experimental studies have shown that children with autism may have a faulty gene that is responsible for breaking down the specific proteins in milk and wheat. For them, accumulation of these proteins in the blood may, in turn, trigger autistic behavior. A protein in cow's milk, casein, is a common food allergen among children with autism, and a growing number of health professionals recommend avoiding cow's milk for this reason as well as the other reasons mentioned in earlier chapters. Gluten, a protein in wheat, also may exacerbate autistic behavior. Your child may benefit from a gluten-free diet.

The last word on diet and behavior has clearly not been written. It will take much more research to nail down the causes of attention deficits, hyperactivity, autistic behavior, and other psychiatric problems. However, a cautious approach is to build your diet from healthy foods as described in chapter 1, avoid food additives and potential allergens to the extent possible, and be guided by your doctor for additional steps that may help.

11

Healthy Eating
for the Young Athlete

Exercise, physical activity, sports—no matter what you call it, moving your body has clear health benefits. Exercise strengthens your heart, improves your metabolism, burns body fat, reduces stress, improves strength and flexibility, and even can increase your life span. Children who grow into an active lifestyle get a wonderful health advantage.

But all that extra activity puts demands on your body. People who exercise have greater energy needs than inactive people, and this is especially true for kids. Fortunately, the guidelines for an active kid's diet are not so different from those for any child. A high-performance diet is made up of a variety of foods from plant sources that are high in carbohydrates, low in fat, and that supply the body with all the nutrients it needs.

Energy from Carbohydrate-Rich Foods

A high-carbohydrate menu is important for everyone, especially active children. "Carbohydrate" means the starchy part of grains, vegetables, or beans. During digestion, it breaks apart to provide natural sugars that are the main fuel for high-intensity work, exercise, or play. Potatoes and other root vegetables, whole grain breads, pastas and other grains, corn, peas, beans, and fruit are great sources of carbohydrates for your child.

When your child gets plenty of high-carbohydrate foods, he or she stores some of the energy in the muscles or liver in special molecules called glycogen, which act like high-energy batteries. When the body is working hard, it depends on these batteries to provide the fuel needed to keep going. One of the key factors in endurance, the ability to continue a given activity for a prolonged period of time, depends on the amount of glycogen stored in your child's muscles. Children can improve their "battery power" by training, getting sufficient rest and energy, and consuming carbohydrate-rich plant foods.

Plant Protein Builds a Healthy Body

Protein is essential for the growth and repair of body tissues. While many people immediately think of meat or eggs, protein found in plants is better for children—and adults, for that matter—in many important ways. On a per-calorie basis, many plant foods have more protein than common animal products. They easily support growth, strength training, and endurance activities without the saturated fat and cholesterol you'll find in meat, poultry, fish, eggs, and dairy products.

From a long-term health perspective, protein from plant sources reduces the risk of chronic illnesses such as diabetes, heart disease, and cancer. In the past, plant proteins were considered to be of "lower quality" than animal proteins because they have a different combination of the same amino-acid building blocks. Some plants have more of one essential amino acid and less of another, while others have the opposite combination. However, when two or more plant proteins are eaten in the same day, these amino acid quantities balance out to make "high quality" proteins used for growth and cell repair. The question of plant protein quality is only an issue for people consuming nearly all of their energy from one food source, such as wheat or rice, day after day, over a prolonged period of time. Luckily, this eating pattern is not typical of most children.

Young athletes can easily get all the protein they need from good-tasting, wholesome food.

A high-performance diet has the following characteristics:

- High in carbohydrates: 65 to 80 percent of calories (mostly *complex* carbohydrates)
  Food sources: grains such as rice, corn, bread, pasta, and cereals; fruit; green vegetables such as beans, broccoli, and spinach; and roots such as potatoes, yams, and carrots.
- Low in fat: 10 to 25 percent of calories (mostly *unsaturated* fat)
  Food sources: nuts, seeds, nut butters, plant oils, beans, and grains.
- Adequate in protein: 10 to 15 percent of calories
  Food sources: beans, nuts, seeds, grains, and vegetables such as spinach, chard, broccoli, and cauliflower.

Adapted from www.newcenturynutrition.com with permission.

The U.S. government's recommendations for protein and calorie intake during childhood are shown on page 117. However, take these recommended levels of protein with a grain of salt. They include a wide safety margin and are higher than is really needed for many children.

Here is what the numbers mean, translated into actual foods: the 16 grams of protein needed by children aged one to three can be found in a cup of soy milk, a package of quick oats, and a slice of bread. A simple menu of breakfast cereal with soy milk (15 grams), a bowl of lentil soup and bread (20 grams), and a serving of spaghetti with marinara sauce and a bowl of corn (13 grams) provides the larger amount of protein needed by teen athletes. The bottom line is that for athletes of any age, it is easy to get the protein needed. See meal planning guidelines in chapters 3 through 8 for more details, and chapters 16 to 18 for recipes and sample menus.

Some people believe that if some protein is good, more must be better. But the truth is, feeding your children extra protein will not make their muscle cells increase in size because protein, by itself, is not a stimulus for muscle growth. The way to increase muscle size and strength is to work the muscles themselves. This same erroneous premise is the motivation behind high-protein weight-

RECOMMENDED DIETARY ALLOWANCES
OF PROTEIN AND CALORIES

SEX AND AGE	AVERAGE GRAMS OF PROTEIN PER DAY	AVERAGE RECOMMENDED CALORIES PER DAY
Girls and boys, 1–3	16	1,300
Girls and boys, 4–6	24	1,800
Girls and boys, 7–10	28	2,000
Girls, 11–14	46	2,200
Boys, 11–14	45	2,500
Girls, 15–18	44	2,200
Boys, 15–18	59	3,300

gain powders and bars marketed to body builders. With advertising slogans such as "Massive, Unequaled Power; Pack on Pound after Pound," these products promise results they cannot deliver.

To make sense out of why more is not better, let's look at how protein is used by the body. Food proteins are like strings of beads, with each "bead" being an amino acid. During digestion, these amino acids come apart, to be used by the body for various purposes. Once we have had enough food protein for the body's needs, the rest is excess. These unneeded amino acids have to be broken down and used for energy or eliminated. In the process, some of the remnants pass through the kidneys, carrying calcium with them. Over time, this loss of calcium is significant, and is one of the biggest contributors to the weakened bones of osteoporosis. Excess protein also strains the kidneys, causing them to gradually lose some of their ability to filter toxins out of your body. When fat and cholesterol come along with all this unneeded protein—which is inevitable with animal products—this extra protein clearly does far more harm than good.

The preferred body fuels are carbohydrates and fats. In short, consuming excess protein is not an efficient way to energize the body or build muscles, and regular high protein intakes increase the risk of chronic disease later.

Keeping Cool

Children are more sensitive than adults to overheating and dehydration. And during vigorous sports, children lose a lot of water through perspiration. The effects of dehydration caused by inadequate fluid intake are rapid and severe. Early signs include cramping, decreased muscle strength and endurance, dry mouth, headache, dizziness, and nausea. Later effects include decreased ability to regulate body temperature, confusion, clumsiness, and loss of consciousness.

Needless to say, your child is focused on winning the game or finishing the hike, not on something as mundane as staying well hydrated. Many children do not stop to drink until they are very thirsty. By the time they do, they are often already dehydrated to some degree. Plain water and other fluids should be readily available to them at all times. Little bottles of water, diluted fruit juices, sports drinks, and even punches are all useful for rehydration, although the use of sugary drinks should be limited to the sport setting. Avoid offering caffeinated or carbonated beverages.

There's nothing like a summer day at the beach or the park. But while many children seem to be able to play for hours in hot weather, they are just as susceptible to the damaging effects of the sun as their adult counterparts. Encourage your child to play in the shade and to take breaks from the hot sun to have a drink of water. Also be sure to lather on sunscreen to prevent sunburn and long-term skin damage.

Children at greatest risk for dehydration are those wearing equipment such as football pads and playing in hot environments, and those limiting water or food intake to lose weight for competitive sports. But these cautions apply to everyone. Even when children are exercising inside or are swimming or playing in water, it's important to have frequent beverage breaks.

Young Bodies and Sports

It's best not to stress weight loss (or gain) or push for change in your child's body shape or size. Because children are growing, their weight and body proportions will change on their own as they mature. Restricting food intake, even in children above healthy weight and fat levels, can have negative effects on growth, exercise performance, concentration, and learning. Instead, serve healthy foods as described in chapter 1 and join your child in exercise and play.

Emphasize that winning the game is not the main goal but that just enjoying it is what's most important. Setting this good example in your life will really help your children feel good about themselves and enjoy being active as they grow into fit, talented adults.

Improving Sports Performance through Diet

Pre-Exercise Meals

Pre-exercise meals are important to ensure that your young athlete has adequate energy to get the most out of his or her activity. There are no magic foods that will guarantee top performance. In sports lore, a lot of focus has been placed on the last meal before exercise, but keep in mind that overall diet has the most important influence on your child's ability to train and compete.

High-carbohydrate foods such as pasta, rice, potatoes, and bread are easily digested and provide readily available fuel. They also help to ward off low blood sugar which can result in light-headedness,

Tips for Kids Competing in Sports

- Two hours before the event or the game, encourage children to eat a nutritious high-carbohydrate, low-fat snack or small meal and to drink at least one cup of water or other beverage.

- After the competition, provide high-carbohydrate foods and fluids to all athletes. Avoid using special food treats to reward winning.

- When you're on the road, pack nutritious food for the competition, because choices available at sporting events are often less than healthy.

- Do not allow a child to deliberately dehydrate to make a weight class in wrestling or other sports.

fatigue, and indecision. The size and type of meal consumed should be related to the amount of time your child has before exercise. Large meals generally take three to four hours to digest; small meals, two to three hours; small snacks and liquids, one to two hours.

While the pre-exercise meal does not contribute immediate energy for exercise, it may be useful if exercise continues for an hour or more. Athletes typically run out of stored carbohydrate after about ninety minutes of exercise, so the pre-competition meal is critical when exercise is prolonged or when a series of shorter competitions occurs over a long period of time, as in a track meet, swim meet, or wrestling tournament.

Many athletes are nervous before competition. A familiar pre-competition meal can help settle the stomach and absorb gastric juices. Athletes who are too nervous to eat before competition need to make a special effort to eat extra food on the previous day, and it is essential that they still drink an adequate amount of fluid. Cool water or a favorite sports drink is usually well tolerated even by a nervous stomach.

When planning your child's pre-exercise meals, don't forget your child's likes and dislikes. Try out new foods during training rather than on an event day.

Eating during Exercise

In events lasting longer than ninety minutes, an energy-containing beverage such as juice, punch, or a sports drink can replenish blood

---

Pre-exercise Meal Timing for Your Child

Morning event/activity	Have a hearty dinner, a bedtime snack, and a small morning snack such as toast and juice.
Afternoon event/activity	Eat a big breakfast and a small lunch.
Evening event/activity	Eat a good breakfast and a hearty lunch and, if time permits, a small snack about two hours before the event.

glucose and extend endurance time. One cup of a dilute sports drink every fifteen minutes provides 25 to 30 grams of carbohydrate and helps ward off dehydration. Easily digested solid foods such as bananas or crackers also work well.

Postexercise Meal

After exhaustive exercise, high-carbohydrate foods are essential for replenishing the muscle's energy stores. Examples include bagels, orange juice, rice, pasta, vegetables, and fruits. If your child is not hungry between events or right after exercise, then juices or sports drinks will do the trick. Bananas and orange juice are potassium-rich and can help replace the electrolytes and minerals that your child has lost through perspiration.

The postexercise meal is most important for children who participate in more than one event at a meet or tournament, or if workouts are prolonged and extensive. Waiting more than two hours to eat after exercise will impair muscle glycogen storage and slow down recovery from strenuous activity.

To replace lost fluids, urge your child to drink until he or she is no longer thirsty, and then have a bit more. Have your child start immediately after exercise, with at least one cup of water or other good-tasting fluid. You can explain that a good way to monitor rehydration is to use the color of urine. Encourage your son or daughter to keep drinking every hour or so until the color of his or her urine has changed from a dark yellow to a pale yellow color.

In this chapter we've covered all the bases—eating during training, before an event, and during recovery—with specifics on foods and amounts. But the fact is, exercise is fun, and fueling it with healthy foods becomes really easy once you get into the groove. Following these simple guidelines will maximize your child's ability to train and compete at his or her best.

12

Nuturing a Healthy
Body Image

Body image issues pervade our lives. How you feel about your body at any given time in your life influences how well you take care of it. It affects what you eat. And, needless to say, it has a dramatic effect on your self-esteem. The same is true for your child and, for that matter, all children. People with distorted or unfavorable body images often limit their participation in social activities and hold themselves back from success in work and their relationships with others, so it is essential to nurture your child to achieve and maintain a healthy body image.

Nurturing a healthy body image is a little tricky, because you and your family are only a few of the many influences on your child. Children learn about body images—desirable or otherwise—from the people they come into contact with and the media messages they hear and see. Many children today have to formulate their body images in a storm of conflicting and potentially damaging influences.

For many, being thin, fit, and beautiful is synonymous with love, success, and power. Physical beauty seems to hold the promise of eternal happiness. Many people believe that if they reach a certain weight or have their nose shape modified, the rest of their lives will fall into place—that somehow it's just one physical characteristic that is keeping them from finding happiness. Many people have a tremendous fear of being too far away from the "ideal."

Sadly, this fear is well founded. "Lookism"—that is, discrimination based on appearance—is alive and well worldwide. Certainly you learn some things about people by outward physical signs—body size and shape, clothing, and hair, for example—that may hint at their exercise and diet habits, income, personality and even perhaps religious affiliation, among others. But people who are large, small, or who have unusual physical features are regularly discriminated against. Studies have shown that people who are heavier than the current "ideal" are less likely to be hired, promoted, given raises, or admitted to top colleges, and they often face discrimination finding housing and health care.

Body image issues can be complicated and far-reaching, ranging from poor self-esteem to eating disorders, steroid use, and beyond. The solutions are somewhat less complicated. An effective strategy, simple as it may sound, is to try to show love for your children unconditionally and valuing them for who they are, rather than placing much stock in how well they traverse the sometimes awkward phases of childhood appearances. Add a bit of guidance for children on how to dress and groom themselves and a solid grounding in healthy eating habits and you've got them started in the right direction.

Parents' feelings toward their children run the gamut from love, admiration, and awe to anger, disappointment, and guilt, and these are all entirely normal. But you have to *show* your child love and support. Show your love through affection, respect, attention—any way you can.

Next, nurturing your children with the healthy foods they need to be slim and strong will provide them with the opportunity to be at their physical best. Adolescent weight worries are likely caused, in part, by meaty, high-fat diets that promote unnecessary weight gain. Talk about nutrition with your children in terms they can understand. By learning about what nutrients do inside their bodies, they will be more likely to eat better food.

In addition to a loving home atmosphere and healthy foods, you can influence your child's body image in three other ways: what you say to or teach your child about his or her body, and how you view and treat your own body, and how you respond to and treat others relative to their body size and shape. What this means is that to nurture a healthy body image for your child, you will need to take a thoughtful look at your feelings about your own body and how that is reflected in how you talk about and treat yourself. In addition, look at how your perceptions of other people's sizes and shapes factor into your responses to them. Children are careful observers. They learn from everything that is going on around them. In the early years especially, they are soaking up the words, ideas, and actions of the people closest to them—you and other family members.

Talking with Your Child

Here are some ideas for nurturing a healthy body image collected from parents, psychologists, students, teachers, and other people who have found them useful.

- Value your children without judgment, just because they are yours. Notice and value their thoughts, abilities, feelings, and qualities. Tell them so. Encourage them to value others in similar ways. Ask questions about your child's feelings or activities.
- Teach your children how to groom themselves and dress well. Avoid overemphasizing the importance of appearance, but don't avoid talking about the basics of self-care either. Send them to school in clean, ironed clothes and, as they get old enough, teach them how to care for their clothes and keep a neat appearance.
- Help your children to understand the wisdom of their bodies and to come to pay attention to its basic needs. A child who can appropriately respond to feelings of hunger, high energy, tiredness, fullness, etc., will be better prepared to make healthy choices throughout life.

- Help your children to understand the purposes of advertising images and why they should not be taken to heart or used to measure personal success.

- Help your children to understand the difference between healthy eating habits (nutrition) and dieting. Encourage healthy eating habits and other lifestyle choices that promote wellness, personal fulfillment, and success. Mealtimes, from preparation to cleanup, can be times for creativity, sharing, and simply enjoying each other's company.

- Listen to the aspirations and goals of your children, and support each of them in their efforts to achieve them.

- Incorporate fun physical activity into your family life. Whether you do it because it feels good, or it's enjoyable, or it's good for your health, you'll want to try new activities and include friends to make exercise a social activity. In the process your children will come to understand both the breadth and the limits of how exercise can influence their body size and shape.

- If your child is dieting, talk to him or her about why he or she wants to lose weight. Be on the lookout for feelings of inadequacy, and deal with those issues. Help your child to understand that skipping meals and cutting calories are not effective over the long run, and to appreciate the connections among healthy eating habits, exercise, body size and shape, and wellness.

- Involve kids in volunteering with people or animals. This shifts their focus away from themselves and onto others who need it more.

You can be a good role model for your children by not criticizing your own body and by eating the same healthy foods that you

Modeling a Healthy Body Image

"You have to make friends with your body, live in it, and trust it."

KAZ COOKE, *REAL GORGEOUS,* 1996

prepare for your children. Don't spend much time talking about physical appearance and diets. You might be surprised how your comments about you and actions affect your child. You'll want to avoid saying things like "I can't eat that, I'm on a diet" or "I hate swimsuit season." Listen to your body's needs for food, rest, and exercise, and take care to meet them.

To refocus on things that matter and away from negative feelings about your own body, you might want to talk instead about thoughts or activities that are most interesting to you or that show care for the people you love. You also may want to notice how easily you accept care, interest, and compliments from others. Finally, if you want to make a lifestyle change, focus on making changes for your health. The result will be your body at its natural best—in form, feeling, and function.

Differences in physical appearance are part of the spice of or interest in life. It is important to avoid criticizing the bodies of others who do not meet your standards of physical beauty. Take a moment to think about the effect your comments might have on the people around you—especially your children. Many adolescents recall specific comments made by their parents, siblings, or friends about the appearance of others and how those comments affected them, sometimes for years. For example, one student decided never to wear shorts again after hearing a family member make a comment about a woman "who had no place wearing shorts in public."

Encouraging other people in your life to lose weight virtually never works. This is especially common among partners when one wishes the other would change his or her body size, shape, or something else about themselves to be more attractive. Situations like this often turn into a battle of wills. Children who observe this may learn the sad lesson that the body is a battleground.

Finally, it helps to think about how we interact with people based upon their body size and shape. Do you treat heavier family members or friends differently than thinner ones? Would you ask your heavier friends to go out to the same type of restaurants or invite them to do the same types of activities as your thinner friends?

The best you can do is love your children like crazy and provide the tools and environment they'll need to shape their own body

The Wrong Assumption?

I still remember the day I realized that I had never asked my stepfather, who had been outside his healthy weight range for many years, to go on a walk or take a hike with me—something I did regularly with other family members. It made me think about other ways I might have been treating him differently, and about how he may have felt, without breathing a word.

AMY JOY LANOU, PH.D.

images. Given all the factors influencing your children, even with your best efforts, it is still possible that they will experience difficulties in achieving and maintaining a healthy body image. It is not your fault. The key is simply to support and encourage your child in his or her efforts to rebuild a healthy body image.

13

Achieving a Healthy Weight and Fitness Level

People come in an amazing range of sizes, shapes, weights, and body styles. A variety of body styles can be healthy and fit. When it comes to health, what counts are your food choices, exercise, relaxation, and work habits as well as tobacco, drug, and alcohol use. When your healthy habits are in place, your healthy form follows.

You will know that your children are fit if they are spending a significant portion of their day in active pursuits and are eating enough healthy foods to meet their energy and nutrient needs. And you'll see the payoff. Achieving a high level of fitness gives them the ability to live life actively, energetically, and fully. Fitness feels good. A fit and rested body is ready to "seize the day." It's ready to take advantage of opportunities and tackle obstacles that come its way.

The Importance of Maintaining a Healthy Weight

People who maintain a healthy weight throughout life are at much less risk of chronic disease and tend to live longer than individuals who are overweight. The factors that are at the root of excess weight—lack of activity and a high-fat diet—also contribute to diabetes, heart disease, high blood pressure, and some cancers. Weight problems are common worldwide, but the United States is leading the way, with 33 percent of adults considered obese and 52 percent of the population considered overweight.

It's not just adults. Children in industrialized countries are getting fatter, too. The prevalence of obesity in nine-year-old children in one recent study published in *Pediatrics,* was about 12 percent for boys and 7 percent for girls in 1994. The number of overweight four-to-five-year-old girls nearly doubled between the early 1970s and the early 1990s. This epidemic goes way beyond cosmetics. Childhood obesity leads to all manner of health problems, such as adult-onset diabetes and heart disease. A number of risk factors for heart disease, stroke, and diabetes, including high blood pressure, high blood cholesterol, and insulin resistance, sometimes are grouped together and called the metabolic syndrome. In one study, published in 1999 in the journal *Annals of Medicine,* obese seven-year-olds had nearly 4½ times the risk of having metabolic syndrome in adulthood than their nonobese peers.

Many overweight children become overweight adults. This is in part because the number of fat cells a child has is determined by the time he or she reaches adolescence. Generally, heavier children have more fat cells, which makes it more difficult for them to lose weight as adults. And sadly, children who are overweight maintain some added health risk even if they eventually lose the weight.

Family plays a major role in determining a child's body size through genetics and environmental influences. Genetics give us our eye and hair color, but when it comes to body size and shape, they are no match for how we live life. Doctors agree that environmental influences mean everything to a child's chances of staying slim and fit. For example, a child with a family history of adult-onset diabetes has double the risk of having diabetes as an adult. However, if the same child remains inactive, eats fatty foods, and becomes obese, he or she has a *fifty times* greater chance of developing diabetes. We are all born with a set of genes, but we can influence how those genes are expressed simply by choosing healthy actions.

For all these reasons, it is important not to wait for your child to grow out of chubbiness, but instead to work with him or her to choose a healthy eating style and incorporate fun physical activity into your lives right away.

What Is a Healthy Weight?

You probably know already if your child is at a healthy weight. But you may wish to check, in the same way doctors do, with what is called the body mass index, or BMI. It's simply a way to look at weight while adjusting for your child's height. To determine BMI, find it in the following table. Then compare your number to the numbers in the table to see if your number lies within the healthy range.

BMI is a simple index of body size. It does not tell you whether extra weight comes from body fat or bulging muscles. In fact, many highly trained, very muscular athletes are heavier than the healthy weight standards, but they usually have a healthy body composition—meaning their "extra" weight is lean muscle mass rather than fat. For most of us, however, maintaining a weight outside of these "norms" is often one of the early signs of a lack of fitness. Check with a medical professional if you have questions about whether your children are above or below their healthy weight.

Food Choices for a Fit Body

Scientists have shown that when people regularly eat low-fat, fiber-rich foods, they achieve and maintain lower weights than when they consume a fat-rich diet. Choosing a plant-based eating style is a simple way to achieve or maintain a healthy weight, because no calorie counting is necessary, and it contains the nutrients a fit body needs. Vegetarians have been shown in numerous studies to be leaner than their meat-eating peers.

FINDING YOUR BMI (KG/M^2)

WEIGHT (POUNDS)	HEIGHT (INCHES)													
	50	52	54	56	58	60	62	64	66	68	70	72	74	76
45	13	12	11	10	9	9								
50	14	13	12	11	10	10	9	9						
55	15	14	13	12	12	11	10	9	9					
60	16	16	15	13	13	12	11	10	10	9				
65	18	17	16	15	14	13	12	11	10	10				
70	20	18	17	16	15	14	13	12	11	11	10			
75	21	20	18	17	16	15	14	13	12	11	11			
80	22	21	19	18	17	16	15	14	13	12	11	11		
85	24	22	21	19	18	17	16	15	14	13	12	12		
90	25	23	22	20	19	18	17	15	14	14	13	12	12	
100	28	26	24	22	21	20	18	17	16	15	14	14	13	12
110	31	29	27	25	23	22	20	19	18	17	16	15	14	13
120	34	31	29	27	25	24	22	20	19	18	17	16	15	15
130	37	34	31	29	27	26	24	22	21	20	19	18	17	16
140	39	36	34	31	29	27	26	24	22	21	20	19	18	17
150	42	39	36	34	31	29	28	26	24	23	21	20	19	18
160	45	42	39	36	34	31	29	27	26	24	23	22	21	19
170	48	44	41	38	36	33	31	29	27	26	24	23	22	21
180	51	47	44	40	38	35	33	31	29	27	26	24	23	22
190		49	46	43	40	37	35	32	31	29	27	26	24	23
200			48	45	42	39	37	34	32	30	29	27	26	24
220				49	46	43	40	38	35	33	31	30	28	27
240					50	47	44	41	39	36	34	33	31	29
260						50	47	44	42	39	37	35	33	32
280								48	45	42	40	38	36	34

Physicians who have encouraged their overweight patients to adopt a plant-based diet have had excellent success in promoting weight loss. Many doctors report that the progression of chronic disease and the need for medications are often reduced. In a study conducted by Hawaiian physician Dr. Terry Shintani, in 1991, patients lost an average of seventeen pounds in three weeks while eating as much food as they wanted. Not surprisingly, the

RECOMMENDED CUTOFF VALUES FOR BMI
(AGES 10–18 YEARS)

| | AT RISK OF OVERWEIGHT | | OVERWEIGHT | |
AGE	MALES	FEMALES	MALES	FEMALES
10	20	20	23	23
11	20	21	24	25
12	21	22	25	26
13	22	23	26	27
14	23	24	27	28
15	24	24	28	29
16	24	25	29	29
17	25	25	29	30
18	26	26	30	30

Source: J. H. Himes and W. H. Dietz. "Guidelines for Overweight in Adolescent Preventive Services: Recommendations from an Expert Committee." *American Journal of Clinical Nutrition* 59 (1994): 307–316.

BMI CLASSIFICATION TABLES FOR ADULTS
(19 YEARS OR OLDER)

BMI CATEGORY	HEALTH RISK	WITH OTHER HEALTH CONDITIONS*
<25	Minimal	Low
25 to <27	Low	Moderate
27 to <30	Moderate	High
>30	High to extremely high	Very high to extremely high

* Such as hypertension, cardiovascular disease, dyslipidemia, Type 2 diabetes, sleep apnea, osteoarthritis, infertility, and other conditions.

Source: www.asbp.org of American Society of Bariatric Physicians.

"Hawaiian" diet was composed mainly of starchy root vegetables, greens, and fruits, similar to the vegan diet discussed in this book. Whatever plant foods you choose, they will be naturally low in fat and encourage a healthy weight.

Dr. Benjamin Spock, pediatrician, medical researcher, and teacher, advised in his book *Dr. Spock's Baby and Child Care* that weight-loss programs for children be based upon changing the *type* of food children eat rather than the *amount* of food they eat. He encouraged shifting the entire family away from oily fried foods, meats, and dairy products and toward low-fat plant based foods— grains, pasta, vegetables, legumes, and fruit. When you do this, he stated, "weight loss typically occurs without anyone going hungry." And this is the key to lifelong weight maintenance.

Most of us were not raised as vegetarians, and the idea of meals without meat may still sound odd to some people. But scientific evidence is clear: The closer your family gets to a pure vegetarian diet, the healthier they'll be. See meal planning guide sections in chapters 1 through 8 for specifics, and chapters 17 and 18 for recipe and menu ideas.

Experiment, and broaden your food options. Try new foods, recipes, and places to eat to keep it interesting and enjoyable. Sometimes when people are changing their food intake because of concerns about health, body size, or personal beliefs, they focus too narrowly on just a small number of foods. Exploring the broad range of healthy foods now available makes a menu change fun, nutritious, and sustainable.

Choose low-fat, nutrient-rich options whenever possible. Try choosing lower-fat recipes and foods. For example, try oven-roasted potatoes instead of French fries, pasta with marinara sauce instead of spaghetti with meatballs, and fruit sorbet instead of ice cream. The net effect is usually a reduction in the number of calories and, of course, fat consumed, in any given portion of food that your child and other family members won't be able to detect. In addition, the introduction of new foods adjusts the taste buds and develops an appreciation for good non-fast-food. Avoid foods and beverages that have lots of energy but few or no nutrients such as candy, soda, punch, cookies, and fried snack foods. Whenever possible, skip the fatty condiments such as creamy salad dressings,

Added Benefits of Choosing a Healthy Eating Style

A few months after I began working at an organization that promotes plant-based eating from a scientific perspective, I had the opportunity to prepare a meal for my coworkers and their significant others. Everyone there had been consuming a plant-based diet for many years—some throughout their lives. When we sat together around a rather large table, I was impressed by several observations. While they ranged in age from thirteen to sixty-something, they each had a slim figure, healthy-looking unblemished skin, and a clear countenance. Each of the adults seemed ageless. One of my colleagues, Bob, who has a son in his thirties, is often mistaken as a person in his thirties himself.

AMY JOY LANOU, PH.D.

mayonnaise, butter, and margarine. Replace meals centered around fatty meats and cheese with those built from grains, legumes, and vegetables. See chapters 16 to 18 for new recipe and menu ideas to help you get started.

Key Steps to Fitness

Fitness has four dimensions: cardiovascular, strength, flexibility, and body composition. Activities that get your heart pumping such as running, swimming, bicycling, aerobics, and playing sports or outdoor neighborhood games improve cardiovascular fitness. Strength-training activities such as weight lifting, push-ups, and sit-ups, as well as many daily tasks such as digging in the garden, lifting boxes, carpentry work, and so forth, improve muscular development and bone strength. Stretching, yoga, gymnastics, dancing, and the martial arts all promote flexibility. A healthy body composition balances muscle and other lean tissue with an appropriate amount of fat tissue for your child's age and sex. Healthy body compositions are achieved through a combination of an active lifestyle and a healthy menu of grains, vegetables, legumes, and fruit.

What if My Child Is Overweight?

Take action now. The first step is to look at your family's lifestyle. The two main contributors to overweight are a low activity level and diets based on meat, dairy, products, and oily foods. Assess your family's eating patterns and activities to determine what changes are needed to promote fitness and achieve healthy weight for you and your family members. The easiest and most effective method is to shift together—all of you, if possible—to a healthier lifestyle. The same healthy habits will benefit you and the rest of your family as well as the child you are concerned about.

Take a "get healthy" approach rather than embarking on a low-calorie diet to achieving fitness and healthy weight. The idea is to focus on *what* you eat, not so much on *quantity*. As you know by now, the healthiest diet avoids animal products completely and is built from grains, legumes, vegetables, and fruits.

Work with your child toward an understanding of food as a fuel for health and fitness rather than as a comfort, friend, enemy, or boredom reliever. Read books to them that present nutrition in a fun and interesting manner. Under most circumstances, restricting the calorie intake of your child is not recommended. Children continue to grow and develop into their early twenties, so you don't want them to be shortchanged of nutrients. It is, however, all right to limit the quantities of snack foods (otherwise known as "empty calorie" foods) and to help your children understand reasonable portion sizes.

Encourage your child to pay attention to his or her natural hunger and fullness cues. Avoid instructing your child "Clean your plate," as he or she may not actually be hungry. We arrive in life with internal signals that keep us from overeating. Try to avoid asking children to override those cues. Instead, help them learn to understand their own feelings of hunger and fullness. If your child does not want to finish his or her meal now, but you are afraid he or she may end up hungry later, simply wrap the plate and save it. Promising dessert as a reward is best avoided as well, as it encourages overeating and makes less healthful foods seem special.

Talk with your child about his or her eating and activity patterns. Look at your child's activities during and after school. How does he or she spend the time between school and dinner? Is he or she eating meals at school? Is your child in physical education class? What does he or she do at recess? If your child's eating or activity patterns seem out of balance, work with him or her to increase activities to at least thirty minutes on most days and to eat three to five healthy meals and snacks a day.

You may want to limit sedentary activities, such as TV watching and computer time, except when homework requires it. It is estimated that, on average, U.S. preschoolers spend twenty-three hours a week in front of the television and grade-school students watch for twenty-nine hours each week. Add to this the time spent playing video games, using the Internet, doing homework, and eating dinner—and you realize that kids are spending a lot of time sitting still.

Encourage your child to play with other children and to do active things with you or another family member. Investigate local organized activity programs in your area and talk to your neighbors about after-school, weekend, and summer activities for kids. Gym class and team sports are not everyone's cup of tea, so encouraging individual interests such as ice skating, ballet dancing, or skateboarding are important, too. In addition to encouraging your child to adopt a healthy, vegetarian eating style, teaching him or her to enjoy being active is likely to be the most important lesson you can offer for your child's long-term health.

Support your school district in its efforts to promote wellness and physical education and to promote healthier lunches in the cafeteria. Many schools are under financial pressure to downsize health and physical education programs. Let school officials know that you think it is important that your child learn life skills that will help support your fitness efforts at home. School lunch programs are required to provide nutritious, low-cost meals to students—you can help them to understand what options you want available for your child.

Staying Clear of the Food Fight

One of the potentially difficult aspects about feeding your family is staying out of the "food fight." The high chair or the dining room table is one of the first places where a child can exert control in his or her life. You or another family member may be the food provider, shopper, or preparer, but the individual diner makes the final decision about whether to eat the food. Children learn very early that what they eat is important to their parents, and children often use this knowledge to their advantage. Have you ever seen a youngster sitting at the table for an hour after dinner while the parents wait for the child to eat one stalk of asparagus? Or have you known a child who is not allowed to eat sweets at home but who chows on cookies at a neighbor's house?

Food also can be used as a reward, a way to exert control, or a way to rebel. Rewards such as "If you get an A on the test, we will stop for ice cream on the way home," or "If you are really good while we shop, you can get a candy bar when we go through the checkout line" are seemingly positive, but they, too, can set up internal conflicts about food. This is especially true if the rewards are in opposition to current goals for health or body image. If not dealt with early, these food fights may extend into adult life as well.

No matter what form the food fight takes, it is full of "shoulds," "shouldn'ts," guilt, and fear. Finding a way to sidestep the food fight is a priority. If your child is having trouble sticking to healthy foods, take a good look at what might be getting in the way. If you find you are already stuck in a food-related conflict, you may want to try some of these strategies to release yourself from these struggles.

Stock up your kitchen with healthy foods. Keeping plenty of fruits, vegetables, grains, and beans on hand and keeping unhealthy foods out of the house is a simple way to eliminate conflict over which type of food to prepare or eat.

Focus on food as a fuel for health. Learn enough to have confidence in your knowledge of nutrition and health. Choose a simple health-giving way of eating like the one suggested in these pages, and explain to your child why it is important to eat this way.

Reduce the emphasis on food in your life. Regularly trying to solve problems by eating or congratulating yourself or your children with food is a sign that the importance of food has gotten out of proportion. Look for other solutions to problems, such as talking about them, writing them in a journal, or taking a walk or a bike ride to figure out some possible solutions. And you can reward yourself or your kids with nonfood treats such as a warm conversation, reading, going to a movie or the park, making something, calling Grandma or a friend, or anything you enjoy doing together.

Set clear divisions of responsibility. If you find yourself in a food fight with your child, clearly define food responsibilities. The parent is responsible for providing appropriate food choices. The child is responsible for choosing what to eat among the choices offered.

Allow for healthy treats. One way to keep from feeling trapped by your healthy eating strategy is to allow both you and your child to have occasional treats. The important thing is to get a new idea about what this means. Try a fresh-fruit smoothie, a colorful cup of berries in season, a vegetable dish prepared a favorite way, or one of the vegan desserts in chapter 18.

The Problem with Dieting

A recent study found that roughly half of American adults are currently trying to lose weight, and adolescent boys are girls are close behind at 36 and 44 percent, respectively. Roughly 20 to 30 percent of dieting adolescents practice an unhealthy or even dangerous diet.

Mothers' Feeding Practices Influence Daughters' Eating and Weight

A recent study from Penn State University provided evidence that dieting and concern for overweight is easily transferred from mother to daughter. The researchers observed that mothers who believed their daughters were at risk of becoming overweight and who were dieting themselves exerted more control over their daughters' eating habits. The daughters responded by becoming heavier, but also more concerned about weight and showed signs of reduced self-control of food intake. Most surprising was the age at which this starts. The maternal food fights were transferred to the *kindergarten-aged* daughters in maternal efforts to protect their daughters from becoming overweight.

In another study of five-to-twelve-year-olds, 45 percent of the girls and 20 percent of the boys reported having been on a diet.

These figures are staggering, especially when you look at the consequences of restricting calories. Cutting calories, while often effective at lowering weight for the short term, usually results in overeating or binge eating and regain of any lost weight. This is a natural antistarvation response to dieting. Caloric restriction alters body chemistry to try to push the dieter to seek out food and makes the body conserve stored energy or hold on to its fat. Some other weight-loss schemes are similarly ineffective or destructive. Diet pills, for example, contain caffeine or other stimulants, laxatives, or diuretics that make you lose water. Crash diets usually leave a person aggravated, discouraged, and the same size.

What if, instead of limiting calories to lose weight, we simply switched to healthy foods? When your diet is built from fruits, vegetables, grains, and legumes, weight management is much easier and putting limits on calories is unnecessary. For example, a veggieburger has 0.5 gram of fat compared to a hamburger at 21 grams, saving 20.5 grams of fat and 180 calories. A bean burrito with lettuce, tomato, and salsa has 3 grams of fat compared to a chili cheese burrito with 14 grams of fat, for a savings of 11 grams of fat and 99 calories. And choosing a pineapple and tomato pizza without the cheese over a pepperoni pizza saves 14 grams of fat per slice and a total of 126 calories! It's easy to make the switch and well worth your time.

When we serve healthy foods and encourage physical activity, our bodies and our children's bodies will find their way to healthy shape and size in a pleasurable and sustainable way.

14

Eating Disorders:
A Guide for Parents

An enormous number of young people fall into a curious relationship with food, a relationship that becomes more and more damaging as time goes on. Seven million American women and one million American men currently suffer from anorexia nervosa or bulimia. It starts early. According to the National Association of Anorexia Nervosa and Associated Disorders, more than one in ten high school students have an eating disorder. Five to 10 percent of obese people have binge-eating disorders. And millions of other young people struggle with their weight, body image, and the consequences of disordered eating habits and activity patterns. Recent studies in Spain, Japan, and China indicate that unhealthy dieting or disordered eating behavior is rising in these countries as well.

It doesn't have to be this way. Our children can be slim and healthy, with a healthy body image. As covered in detail in chapters 12 and 13, choosing a plant-based eating style and an active lifestyle are the best places to start. But even in families with the best intentions, children sometimes get caught in self-destructive patterns and dissatisfaction with their bodies. These problems have multiple causes. Often they are motivated by the child's need for control in his or her life, or are coping mechanisms for dealing with difficult situations. The good news is that eating disorders usually are treatable when you know the warning signs and where to turn for help.

The Unhealthy Habits

Disordered eating habits come in three basic types: restriction, overeating, and purging. Each takes a variety of forms, and some can be quite difficult to differentiate from normal behavior.

Restriction. This is characterized by dieting—that is, limiting food intake, starvation, use of appetite suppressants, or skipping meals for weight loss. Just to be clear, changing one's eating choices to include more healthy foods (or to avoid animal products or junk food) is not an eating disorder, and should not be considered "restriction" in this sense.

Overeating. This means binge eating, regularly eating beyond fullness, constant eating, or simply consuming more food than you need.

Purging. This includes the use of over-the-counter drugs such as emetics to stimulate vomiting, laxatives to induce diarrhea, or diuretics to stimulate the loss of fluids. Other methods used to "purge" the body of energy and/or weight include exercising excessively, spitting chewed food back out before swallowing, and purposeful dehydration through sweating or limiting fluid intake.

Often all three problems can occur in the same person at different times. Disordered eating or activity usually is a sign that something is not right in a child's life. Sometimes the solution is as simple as learning more about healthy ways to lose weight, or appropriate portion sizes. Everyone wants to enjoy food, but young people may not realize how the fat content in burgers, fries, and chicken nuggets is so easily turned to excess body fat. With a little guidance you can show them which foods won't betray their bodies. In the process you could prevent a serious disorder. However, sometimes the solution is more complicated and goes way beyond food. If you notice that your child has troubled eating habits or excessively exercises, seek help as soon as possible. The solutions are simpler and quicker when put to early use.

The Dangers of Eating Disorders

Here are some of the physical consequences of disordered eating and activity.

- Restrictive dieting and skipping meals sometimes result in weight loss in the short term, but they spark a cycle of problems. Restricting the amount you eat will inevitably make you hungry and overly focused on food. Eventually your willpower will fold, so you'll then overeat, feel guilty, gain weight back, and get discouraged. Like it or not, this cycle is the result of your natural biology. When you deprive your body of food, your body responds by insistently asking for it. So the natural biological consequence of restriction is overeating—it is not due to a "lack of willpower."

- Starvation, or severe food restriction, has very serious consequences—weakness; growth failure; severe nutritional deficiencies; irregular heartbeat and weakening of heart and other organs; premature bone loss; hair loss; dry, blotchy skin; lack of energy; infertility; insomnia; and even death.

- Diet pills, or appetite suppressants, usually are not effective for a person who is restricting intake, because the strong physiological response to dieting overrides the weak effects of these drugs. Most over-the-counter brands contain stimulants such as caffeine, diuretics that cause water loss, or some type of fiber to slow the emptying of food from the stomach and contribute to a feeling of fullness.

- Binge eating causes bloating, discomfort, and usually weight gain. Binges can range from about a thousand to more than ten thousand calories and usually are made up of high-fat, high-sugar, and sometimes salty foods. The result is nutritional imbalances, and severe binges have been known to cause stomach rupture.

- Overeating usually causes weight and fat gain.

- Vomiting, when induced regularly, causes serious problems, including swollen glands in the face and neck, severe tooth decay, reddened eyes, bloating, fatigue, dehydration, urinary tract infections, torn or damaged throat and esophagus, chronic heartburn, and even heart failure due to potassium depletion.

- Dehydration using pills or other methods, including purging, can result in very dangerous consequences: frequent urinary tract infections, morning headaches, bloating, sensitivity to heat, loss of muscle strength and endurance, mental confusion, kidney stones, heat stroke, and death.

- Laxatives are ineffective at removing calories (only an estimated 10% of calories eaten are lost) and cause discomfort, dehydration, and electrolyte and nutrient imbalances. A colon that is regularly attacked with laxatives begins to depend on them to work at all and requires higher and higher doses to get the "desired" effect. Long-term use can permanently damage the colon.

- Exercise, within limits, is healthy. But when taken to excess, exercise, too, can have harmful consequences, such as muscle, tendon, or bone injury; lack of energy caused by overtraining; frequent illness; or dehydration.

Anorexia Nervosa

Anorexia nervosa is, in essence, self-starvation. Although the word "anorexia" literally means "lack of appetite," the truth is that most people with anorexia are almost always hungry. They work to control their hunger by extreme dieting and rigid exercise regimens, often ending up emaciated. Anorexia can be life-threatening and very difficult to treat. Some 20 percent of individuals with anorexia never recover.

Physicians use the following guidelines to diagnose anorexia nervosa:

- loss of 25 percent or more of body weight and refusal to maintain healthy body weight
- intense fear of gaining weight
- perception of self as overweight, despite extreme thinness
- in women, the absence of at least three consecutive menstrual cycles

Ninety percent of those with anorexia nervosa are female, often in their teenage years. Studies show that girls are falling into anorexia at younger and younger ages, reflecting the increasing number of preteens who are either on diets or concerned about their weight. Many excel in academics and after-school activities, and they are often perfectionists or overachievers. Their families often pressure them to excel.

Bulimia Nervosa

More common than anorexia, bulimia nervosa is characterized by binge eating followed by attempts to get rid of the food. The word "bulimia" means "hunger of an ox," which is not a bad description, given that a binge could include what another person would eat over an entire day, or even a week. A doctor will diagnose bulimia when binges happen at least twice a week for three months and are regularly followed by any type of purging, such as self-induced vomiting, laxative abuse, the use of diuretics or enemas, extended periods of fasting, or excessive exercise.

People with bulimia often feel a lack of control during binges and are persistently concerned with body weight and shape. However, many are at their normal weight, which often helps to conceal their condition and delays medical attention. The results can be very serious, even life-threatening.

Athletes or others with weight requirements, such as wrestlers, dancers, and gymnasts, are at particular risk of bulimia. Not surprisingly, it is especially common in the teenage and young adult years. In some studies, up to a third of college women regularly binge and purge to control their weight.

Binge-Eating Disorder

Binge eating is the most common of all the eating disorders. In a survey of college women, one in five said they binge eat. The term "binge-eating disorder" was introduced in 1992 to replace the terms "compulsive overeating," "emotional overeating," and "food addiction." Unlike bulimia nervosa, binge-eating disorder does not involve purging or other attempts to eliminate food. Binge eaters often feel disgusted, guilty, and depressed after overeating, but also feel powerless to control their behavior.

About half of binge eaters are overweight. Some manage to maintain their weight in a normal range by restricting calorie intake between binges. Binge-eating disorder affects men and women from all races and in all age groups. It is not limited to adolescents and young adults, as anorexia and bulimia usually are. Often, compulsive overeaters binge to escape loneliness, boredom, or depression. Seeking professional help can be the first step to recovery and wellness.

Activity Disorders

Activity disorders are similar to eating disorders. Compulsive exercisers work out for long periods and have difficulty stopping. They may get up in the middle of the night to exercise or stay on an exercise machine for hours and hours. Some are motivated by fear of gaining weight. For others, exercise has become an addiction. As a result of incessant exercise, they are often underweight, even though they may eat a normal amount of food.

Beyond Definitions

Understanding eating disorders is much more complex than just learning their definitions. Something deeper than food issues or body dissatisfaction is bothering the individual, and he or she has funneled these negative emotions into disordered habits as a way of coping. Most are not fully aware of the emotions fueling their actions. But they often have low self-esteem, feelings of emptiness, feelings of helplessness, and a strong desire for respect and admiration. Eating-disordered teens also may want to be perfect, may have difficulty expressing their feelings, and may be distrustful of themselves and others. They often lack the skills for more constructive methods of coping.

You may be asking yourself: Aren't these feelings normal for children and teens? The answer is yes, kids often experience troubling feelings. The problem lies in how the child deals with them. If you are wondering whether you should be concerned about your child's eating habits, activity patterns, and body image, here is what to look for. If your child has three or more of the following warning signs, you have reason for concern.

- being preoccupied with food and weight
- counting calories or fat grams in all foods
- disappearing into the bathroom after meals

- missing food and/or evidence of secretive eating
- exercising excessively
- constant looking in the mirror and asking how clothes fit
- avoiding mealtimes
- complaining of being fat, or of specific body parts being too fat
- taking an extremely long time to eat, or cutting food in tiny pieces
- constantly talking about the latest diet or new recipes
- eating only fat-free, sugar-free, and other diet foods
- overusing laxatives, diuretics, enemas, diet pills, or other stimulant drugs
- drinking large amounts of coffee and other caffeine-containing beverages
- skipping meals and eating sweets instead
- expressing guilt after eating

If Your Child Has an Eating Disorder

The most important thing you can do is listen to your child. Children with eating disorders feel very alone and find it painful to talk about what they are feeling. Try to be understanding, and try not to argue, accuse, or criticize. Simply express your concern, report what you have observed, and encourage him or her to see a professional with you or on his or her own. Offering your ear and unconditional love and support can provide the strength your child needs to seek further assistance.

Do not try to treat your child yourself. Only an experienced therapist or doctor can treat eating disorders effectively, as they are complex and challenging. If your child is reluctant to get help, you may need to contact therapists or support groups in your area for strategies and suggestions. Eating disorders pose a great emotional and physical threat and should not be left untreated. Unfortunately, eating disorders rarely respond to a quick fix—recovery usually requires help, patience, and a commitment to getting well.

It is important to avoid thinking of eating disorders as a failure in parenting. Many of the factors that contribute to eating disorders are beyond your control. The fact is, you have done your child a great favor by recognizing an eating disorder and helping him or her to seek treatment. Even so, the situation can be taxing on you and the rest of the family, so be sure you take care of yourself in the process of getting help for your child. Aside from listening to, supporting, and offering unconditional love to your child, there isn't a lot you can do; most of the hard work has to come from the person with the disorder.

Finding Appropriate Treatment

Depending on how serious the eating disorder is and how long your child has been struggling with it, there are different treatment options available. Getting your child to agree to meet with an experienced therapist is a good place to start. The therapist can help you and your child evaluate the level of care needed. For some, support groups through community centers, churches, and local colleges are effective. Overeaters Anonymous and Eating Addicts Anonymous are two groups that take a supportive approach to recovery. Check your phone book for local groups. Sometimes individual outpatient therapy with an experienced psychologist, in combination with support groups, is the winning combination.

Many young adults recover from eating disorders through outpatient treatment. Some of the best programs have an integrated treatment team, including a psychiatrist, psychotherapist, dietitian, family physician, and sometimes an exercise physiologist. The psychiatrist may prescribe medications such as antidepressants and anti-anxiety drugs. The psychotherapist will help the child understand feelings and relationships. The nutritionist will look at the child's diet and eating patterns, while the family physician will keep an eye on the child's general health.

Some eating disorders are too serious to be treated by outpatient therapy and require hospitalization or treatment at a residential facility. This is common when there is severe weight loss or gain; inability to carry out normal daily activities; failure of outpatient treatment; or medical problems such as a heart abnormality, dehydration, or very low pulse and blood pressure. If a child mentions suicide, even if only briefly or jokingly, there may be need for hospitalization. Many hospitals and residential treatment facilities now

Looking for a Therapist?

It is perfectly reasonable to "shop" for the best therapist for your child. Here are some questions you may want to ask:

1. What training and experience do you have in treating eating disorders?

2. What is your treatment approach?

3. Do you work with other professionals as part of a treatment team?

4. What are your opinions about medication?

5. How do you gauge success?

offer comprehensive care for eating disorders. A detailed list of centers is found in *The Eating Disorder Sourcebook* by Carolyn Costin (Los Angeles: Lowell House, 1997).

The Internet also may be a useful resource. The National Association of Anorexia Nervosa and Associated Disorders has a useful Web site (www.anad.org), or call their hotline number, 847-831-3438. Also valuable are the Eating Disorders referral site (www.edreferral.com), and the site for Anorexia Nervosa and Related Eating Disorders (www.anred.com).

Often one of the most difficult aspects of treatment is convincing the person with the eating disorder to accept help. Some common barriers include fear of asking for help; lack of clarity on how to ask for it; or, perhaps most damagingly, a belief that he or she does not deserve help. Unfortunately, many victims reach life-threatening situations before they are ready to accept help. Real recovery begins when the individual really wants to get better.

A Few Things to Avoid

Don't try to force a person with an eating disorder to eat. When family and friends "encourage" or force someone to eat—even when it is out of concern and love—these actions will leave the person feeling scolded and out of control. This is not helpful. Eating-disordered individuals already suffer from crushing guilt over their feelings and actions, especially eating. If your child needs to be force-fed to save his or her life, leave that to medical personnel.

Instead, do your best to keep the lines of communication open. Talking with your child in a loving manner and trying to understand his or her feelings are much more helpful. Avoid angry, manipulative, or controlling statements. While these statements may be good ways to air your frustration, they do not aid in the child's recovery.

Avoid negatively commenting on body size and shape with things such as "You look like a concentration camp victim," "Are you sick?," or "What's with all the weight loss?" These comments only perpetuate low self-esteem. Controlling statements such as "Would you just eat already?" and "You had better not go running again after dinner!" and manipulative ones such as "Why are you doing this to me?" also are problematic for a child with an eating disorder. If your relationship is good, a gentle "Would you like to share a meal with me?" or "Please talk to me about what's going on" is much more effective. It is always okay to approach a child with a caring statement such as "It seems as if you've lost a lot of weight, and I'm concerned about you," followed with an offer to listen.

What Can We Expect during Recovery?

Recovery is a long process. Some people struggle with their relationship with food and weight for their whole lifetime, passing from denial to fear, anger, impatience, hope, and acceptance. Some recover in a few months and lead healthy lives unencumbered by disordered eating habits. Most will be conscious of eating habits and body image throughout their lives.

Only about half of people with eating disorders recover fully. Most recover partially, and, unfortunately, some do not survive. The good news is that the prognosis is much better when the eating disorder is caught early. You can help your child by watching out for disordered eating behaviors, helping him or her seek treatment if necessary, and offering your continual love and support throughout the recovery process.

15

Putting It All Together

Our kids have advantages no other generation has had. They can profit from an impressive body of medical research that has matured over many decades, guiding their pediatricians—and their families—toward the most healthful possible diets.

We now know how to prevent, at least to a substantial degree, most of the diseases that have been major killers up to now. While their grandparents may have thought that heart disease was an inevitable part of getting older, children today can virtually sidestep it with wise diet and lifestyle choices. We have learned how to cut the risk of many forms of cancer. Stroke, diabetes, and hypertension can all be held at arm's length by preventive steps that were only dimly understood a generation ago.

As children reach adulthood, they can take advantage of instant access to virtually unlimited health information via the electronic media. Whereas once research studies gathered dust in medical libraries, today they can be read immediately by anyone.

And healthy foods are more available than ever. With more and more movement of people to and from other lands, a kid in Idaho thinks nothing of having lunch of foods from Mexico and dinner from China, while Dad and Mom can practice their Italian or Thai cooking skills.

Even so, our kids have risks that no other generation has had. A few decades ago, fast foods, snack vending machines, and convenience stores were uncommon. Today they are everywhere. School lunch programs serve unhealthy foods, catering more to meat and dairy purveyors than to children's health needs. Exercise is rapidly becoming a thing of the past as television and computers rivet children to their chairs for hours on end and as cars replace walking and bikes and the primary mode of transportation.

The result is that despite our being having better health information than ever before, our kids are more out of shape than at any time in our history. More children than ever are overweight. The artery changes that will one day cause heart disease start before they graduate from high school. The poor nutritional habits many kids learn today are sowing the seeds of cancer, diabetes, and hypertension that will arrive all too soon. Their doctors, ever pressed to dispense prescriptions to try to cope with these burgeoning problems, are likely to fumble with questions about the nutritional steps that could be much more decisive.

You now hold in your hands the opportunity to change this scenario. By serving foods that keep your children healthy, you are doing them a tremendous favor. And the healthy habits they learn will help insulate them, at least a bit, from the seductive but unhealthy foods they'll find all around them.

And you'll be doing them an even bigger favor by joining them in healthy eating habits. As much as they need good health themselves, they also need healthy parents who will be part of their lives for many years to come. They'll profit from your wisdom as they plan their own families and wrestle with the challenges of modern life, including the question of how best to nourish *their* children.

We hope you have found the information in this book helpful, and we wish the very best of health and success to you and your children.

16

Cooking Tips
and Techniques

This section includes recipes, menus, and tips for preparing delicious and healthful meals for your family. It begins with practical suggestions for menu planning and shopping, including sample menus that will be sure to please hungry children. "Stocking Your Pantry" provides suggestions for staple ingredients as well as convenient instant meals to keep on hand, and the Glossary lists foods that may be new to you. The recipes are quick and easy to prepare, with ingredients that are available in most grocery stores. You'll find healthful versions of familiar foods as well as some recipes for experimenting with new flavors. Each of the recipes includes a nutrient analysis to help you choose menus appropriate to your family members' nutritional needs.

Planning a Menu

Planning ahead is the key to easy meal preparation. You'll be amazed at the time and money you save by planning weekly menus and shopping for a week at a time. When you plan ahead you save time looking for parking and standing in line, and you spend less money on impulse items and instant meals. With a busy schedule, having all the ingredients you need on hand when you are ready to make a meal makes eating healthfully at home enjoyable.

Set aside a bit of time and find a quiet spot to plan a one-week menu. Your menu plan does not need to specify every item for every meal. Do think about and include fruit and vegetable favorites of your family members. Over the course of the week be sure to have something that each person will especially enjoy. Breakfasts, especially during the week, probably will be much the same from day to day: fruits, whole grain cereals, and breads. You may want to plan a special breakfast or a cook-together with your children for one weekend morning when you have a little more time.

For lunches, soup (either homemade or commercially prepared) is a quick and nutritious option. Add whole grain bread and salad mix sprinkled with seasoned rice vinegar for a feast in minutes. Children often enjoy "fun" foods such as sloppy joes or pinwheels. Leftovers make perfect instant meals. Serve "sloppy" reheated leftovers over a whole wheat bun, or wrap mashed beans or a dip on a tortilla, add grated carrots and lettuce, roll tightly, and slice to make a colorful pinwheel. Bean or grain salads also are excellent lunch foods that can be prepared in quantity and kept on hand for a quick meal. For many people a weekly lunch menu plan will include a couple of soups and two or three salads.

For dinners, plan four main dishes, prepared in large enough quantities to provide at least two meals for your family. Add whole grains, such as brown rice or bulgur wheat, and vegetables for complete, satisfying meals. Choose vegetables that will offer a variety of color and nutrients, and plan make-ahead foods for nights when you or other family members may not be home in time to cook.

A Sample Menu Plan

This flexible menu plan doesn't specify exact meals for each day of the week. The indicated meals can be prepared according to your time and taste. At the same time, it provides you with the assurance that the ingredients for any of the meals will be available when you need them. Use this menu plan to make a shopping list.

SAMPLE MENU PLAN

Breakfasts

 fresh fruit: strawberries, cantaloupe, oranges, bananas

 toast: whole wheat raisin, multigrain

 hot cereal: oatmeal, 10-grain cereal, cracked wheat

 cold cereal: shredded wheat, Maple Walnut Granola

 French Toast, Polenta

Lunches

 soups: Split Pea Soup, Potato Vegetable Soup, Alphabet Soup

 salads: Chinese Noodle Salad, Three Bean Salad, Potato Salad

Dinners

 Very Primo Pasta

 Crispy Green Salad

 Tamale Pie

 Broccoli with Golden Sunshine Sauce

 Yves Veggie Cuisine Burgers

 Oven Fries

 Garlicky Green Beans

 Sloppy Joes

 Lentil Barley Stew

 Rainbow Salad

Making a Shopping List

Use your menu plan to create a shopping list. Look up the recipes you've chosen and note the ingredients you'll need to purchase. Add fresh vegetables and fruits, whole grains and breads to round out your meals. Check the refrigerator, freezer, and pantry to see what staples need to be restocked (see "Stocking Your Pantry" on page 158). These might include frozen foods, canned foods, condiments, spices, and easy-to-add-to-the-lunch-box items such as single-serve applesauce or other "packables," and beverages.

 To streamline your shopping trip, arrange the foods on your list in categories that reflect the departments in your grocery store, such as fresh produce, grains, dried beans, canned fruits and vegetables, and frozen foods.

SAMPLE SHOPPING LIST

Fresh Produce

oranges	celery	broccoli
bananas	sweet potatoes	zucchini
cantaloupes	green onions	avocados
strawberries	red bell peppers	yellow onions
other seasonal fruits	tomatoes	red onions
	mushrooms	garlic
prewashed salad mix	green cabbage	other seasonal vegetables
	red cabbage	
carrots	potatoes	

Breakfast Cereals

oatmeal	shredded wheat	10-grain cereal

Grains and Pasta

rolled oats	polenta	cornmeal
hulled barley	whole wheat pastry flour	elbow macaroni
brown basmati rice		alphabet pasta

Dried Beans, Peas, and Nuts

lentils	split peas	walnuts

Canned Vegetables and Fruits

28-ounce can crushed tomatoes	roasted red peppers	Single-serve applesauce or fruit cups (packed in juice)
15-ounce can kidney beans	15-ounce can vegetarian chili beans	

Packaged Foods

ramen soups	fortified soy milk or rice milk	maple syrup

Refrigerated Foods

tofu   flour tortillas

Bread

whole wheat bread   whole wheat
burger buns

Vinegar and Condiments

reduced-sodium   balsamic vinegar
soy sauce

Herbs and Spices

chili powder   oregano

Frozen Foods

veggieburgers   apple juice   chopped spinach
orange juice   concentrate
concentrate

You will notice that the shopping list specifies *seasonal* fruits and vegetables. This refers to items that are fresh and in season— for example, tomatoes and peppers in late summer and fall, and citrus fruits in winter and spring. Fruits and vegetables that are in season cost less, have better flavor, and are more nutritious than those that are not in season. Local farmers' markets sell mostly seasonal products, and many stores feature seasonal produce in their advertising flyers and store displays.

Stocking Up

With your shopping list in hand, you'll be ready to stock up quickly and conveniently for the whole week. Make sure you've eaten *before* you head for the store. Shopping on an empty stomach can override the best of intentions and lead to impulsive purchases of less-than-nutritious foods.

Most processed foods have nutrition labels and ingredient lists that provide you with useful information for making healthy food choices. The nutrition label indicates the size of a single serving and the number of calories as well as the amount of fat, protein, sugar, fiber, and salt in that serving. You can also gather useful information by reading through the ingredients list. Listed in order of prominence in the food, the ingredient present in the greatest amount is first on the list, and so forth. Thus, if fat or sugar appears near the top of the list, you know that these are major ingredients. The ingredients list is handy for identifying the presence of artificial flavors, artificial colors, preservatives, and other additives you may wish to avoid.

As you read through the ingredients list, be aware of the many different forms of sugar that may be in food. Sucrose, fructose, dextrose, corn syrup, honey, and malt are just a few, and in general, any ingredients that end with "ose" are sugars. If a product contains several different types of sugar it is likely that sugar is a major ingredient, even if it isn't the first item on the list.

You will also want to avoid foods that contain hydrogenated oils. These oils have been processed to make them solid, or saturated, and like other saturated fats, they can raise blood cholesterol levels and increase the risk of heart disease.

When choosing cereals or soy or rice milks, look for ones that are fortified with calcium, vitamin D, and vitamin B_{12}. Fortified foods from plant sources make getting enough of these nutrients easier. Many brands of orange, grapefruit, and apple juice, both fresh and frozen concentrate types, are now fortified with calcium as well. In addition to the beans and dark, leafy green vegetables, these foods can significantly add to your child's intake of this important nutrient.

Some food products may contain specific nutrition claims, such as "fat-free," "low cholesterol," or "lite." The definitions of these terms, as outlined by the U.S. Food and Drug Administration, are given in the following list.

Light (lite). May refer to calories, fat, or sodium. Contains a third fewer calories, or no more than half the fat of the higher-calorie, higher-fat version; or no more than half the sodium of the higher-sodium version.

Calorie-free. Contains fewer than 5 calories per serving.

Fat-free. Contains fewer than 0.5 gram of fat per serving.

Low-fat. Contains 3 grams (or less) of fat per serving.

Reduced or less fat. At least 25 percent less fat per serving than the higher-fat version.

Cholesterol-free. Contains fewer than 2 milligrams of cholesterol and 2 grams (or less) of saturated fat per serving.

Low cholesterol. Contains 20 milligrams (or less) of cholesterol and 2 grams (or less) of saturated fat per serving.

Reduced cholesterol. At least 25 percent less cholesterol than the higher-cholesterol version and 2 grams (or less) or saturated fat per serving.

Sodium-free. Contains fewer than 5 milligrams of sodium per serving and no sodium chloride in ingredients.

Very low sodium. Contains 35 milligrams (or less) of sodium per serving.

Low sodium. Contains 140 milligrams (or less) of sodium per serving.

Stocking Your Pantry

BASIC INGREDIENTS AND QUICK FOODS

Produce

yellow onions	baby carrots	kale or collard
red onions	celery	greens
garlic	prewashed salad	apples
red potatoes	mix	oranges
russet potatoes	prewashed spinach	bananas
green cabbage	broccoli	

Grains and Grain Products

short-grain brown rice	whole wheat pastry flour	whole wheat couscous
long-grain brown rice	unbleached flour	rolled oats
	potato flour	polenta
bulgur	rice flour	cornmeal
whole wheat flour	barley flour	eggless pasta

cold breakfast
cereals without
added fat or
sugars

hot breakfast
cereals

Dried Beans, Lentils, and Peas

pinto beans

black beans

lentils

split peas

black bean flakes:
Fantastic Foods,
Taste Adventure

pinto bean flakes:
Fantastic Foods,
Taste Adventure

Canned Foods

basic beans (pinto,
garbanzo, kidney,
black)

prepared beans
(vegetarian chili,
baked beans,
refried beans)

tomato products
(crushed toma-
toes, tomato
sauce, tomato
paste)

vegetables (corn,
beets, water-
packed roasted
red peppers)

vegetarian soups

vegetarian pasta
sauce (preferably
fat-free)

salsa

Frozen Foods

unsweetened juice
concentrates
(apple, orange,
white grape)

frozen bananas

frozen berries

frozen vegetables
(corn, peas,
Italian green
beans, broccoli)

chopped onions

frozen diced bell
peppers

Nuts, Seeds, and Dried Fruit

peanut butter

tahini (sesame
seed butter)

raisins

Breads, Crackers, and Snack Foods

whole grain bread
(may be frozen)

whole wheat pita
bread

corn tortillas (may
be frozen)

whole wheat
tortillas (may be
frozen)

fat-free snack
foods (crackers,
rice cakes, pop-
corn cakes, baked
tortilla chips,
pretzels)

Convenience Foods

vegetarian ramen and soup cups

silken tofu

vegetarian burgers, cold cuts, hotdogs

baked tofu

textured vegetable protein

Condiments and Seasonings

herbs and spices

reduced-sodium soy sauce

cider vinegar

balsamic vinegar

seasoned rice vinegar

vegetable broth

vegetable oil spray

molasses

maple syrup

raw or turbinado sugar

baking soda

low-sodium baking powder (Feather-weight)

spreadable fruit

fat-free salad dressing

eggless mayon-naise (Vegenaise, Nayonaise)

stone-ground mustard

catsup

Beverages

fortified soy milk or rice milk

frozen concentrate juice and juice boxes

Meal Preparation Timesavers

With your menu and ingredients on hand, you will be able to pre-pare satisfying meals quickly and conveniently. You may wish to block off a slightly larger period of time and prepare several different menu items in a single cooking session as a further timesaver.

If you have a toddler and have hit on a small selection of coveted foods, you may want to make enough for several days. You will notice that most of the recipes in this book provide six to eight serv-ings. As a result, you will probably have food left over that can be used to provide one or more extra meals. In this way the menu you create may provide meals for more than a week, with no additional shopping, planning, or cooking.

Another timesaver is to make slight modifications to the food you've already prepared so it has a different appearance the second or third time you serve it. In this way you can have maximum variety with a minimum of preparation. The Quick Chili Beans (see page 209) are a good example. Start out by preparing a double batch and serve it as chili with cornbread or over rice. For a second meal, cook it down a little to thicken it, and serve it as a burrito filling or as a baked potato topping. Or layer it in a casserole pan with tortillas, rice, corn, and sautéed zucchini and mushrooms, bake until it bubbles, and call it stacked enchiladas.

Foods that take a bit of time to cook can be prepared in large enough quantities to provide for several meals. Brown rice is a good example. Once cooked, it can easily be reheated in a microwave or on the stovetop and served as a side dish with a variety of recipes. It also can be added to soups and stews, or used as a filling in a burrito or a wrap. Even other hearty grains such as Multigrain Cereal (see page 175) can be made in a large batch on Sunday morning, then reheated and decorated with your child's favorite fresh and dried fruit and stirred up with a bit of cinnamon and soy milk.

Cooking Techniques

Vegetables

The secret to preparing vegetables is to cook them only a much as is needed to tenderize them and bring out their best flavor. The following methods are quick and easy and enhance the flavor and texture of vegetables.

Steaming. A collapsible steamer rack can turn any pot into a vegetable steamer. Heat about 1 inch of water in a pot. Arrange the prepared vegetables in a single layer on a steamer rack and place them in the pot over the boiling water. Cover the pot with a lid and cook until just tender. Sweet potatoes; snow peas; asparagus; and soft, leafy greens are especially appealing cooked this way.

Braising. This technique is identical to sautéing, except that a fat-free liquid is used in place of oil. It is particularly useful for mellowing the flavor of vegetables such as onions and garlic. Heat approximately ½ cup of water, vegetable broth, or wine (the liquid you use will depend on the recipe) in a large pan or skillet. Add the vegetables and cook over high heat, stirring occasionally, adding small amounts of additional liquid if needed, until the vegetables are tender. This will take about five minutes for onions. Braising is a great method for cooking mushrooms, onions, collards, kale, zucchini, green beans, and carrots.

Grilling. High heat seals in the flavors of vegetables and adds its own distinctive flavor as well. Vegetables can be grilled on a barbecue or electric grill, or on the stove using a nonstick grill pan. Cut all the foods that will be grilled together into a uniform size. Preheat the grill, then, add the vegetables. Cook over medium-high heat, turning occasionally with a spatula until uniformly browned and tender. Vegetables that are easily managed with tongs are great on the grill. Large mushrooms, corn on the cob, asparagus, sliced eggplant, sliced squash, and quartered sweet peppers are good examples.

Roasting. A simple and delicious way to prepare vegetables is to roast them in a very hot oven (450°F). Toss the vegetables with seasonings and a small amount of olive oil if desired. Spread them in a single layer on a baking sheet and place them in the preheated oven until tender.

Microwave. A microwave oven provides an easy method for cooking vegetables, particularly those that take a long time to cook with other methods. Another benefit of microwave cooking for vegetables is that they cook quickly with little or no water, minimizing loss of nutrients. Try the recipes for potatoes, sweet potatoes, yams, and winter squash on page 214.

Grains

Whole grains are a mainstay of a healthy diet. The term "whole grain" refers to grains that have been minimally processed, leaving the bran and germ intact. As a result, whole grains provide significantly more nutrients, including protein, vitamins, and minerals, than refined grains. In addition, whole grains are an excellent source of fiber. Grains tend to have mild flavors that are appealing to young and older palates alike. Some fairly common whole grains include whole wheat berries, cracked wheat and bulgur, whole wheat flour, brown rice, rolled oats, whole barley, and barley flour. Some of the less common grains that are slowly making their way into the mainstream are quinoa ("keen-wah"), amaranth, kamut ("kam-oo"), and teff.

Grains should be stored in a cool, dry location. If the outer bran layer has been disturbed by crushing or grinding, as happens in making flour or rolled oats, the grain should be used within two to three months. Properly stored grains with the outer bran layer intact remain viable and nutritious for several years.

When cooking grains, the following tips are useful.

- The easiest way to cook most grains is to simmer them, loosely covered, on the stovetop.
- Lightly roasting grains in a dry skillet before cooking enhances their nutty flavor and gives them a lighter texture. The flavor of millet is particularly enhanced by roasting.
- Grains should not be stirred during cooking, unless the recipe indicates otherwise. They will be lighter and fluffier if left alone.
- When cooking grains, make enough for several meals. Cooked grains can be reheated in a microwave or on the stovetop.
- An easy way to reheat grains on the stove is to place them in a vegetable steamer over boiling water.
- Fine-textured grains such as couscous and bulgur are actually fluffier when they are not cooked. Simply pour boiling water over the grain, then cover and let stand for fifteen to twenty minutes. Fluff the grain with a fork before serving.

Legumes

The term "legume" refers to dried beans and peas such as soybeans, black beans, pinto beans, garbanzos or chickpeas, lentils, and split peas. Legumes may be purchased dried, canned, and in some cases, frozen or dehydrated. Dried beans are inexpensive and easy to cook. If you don't have the time to cook dried beans, canned beans are a good alternative. Kidney beans, garbanzo beans, pinto beans, black beans, and many others are available, including some in low-sodium varieties. For an even quicker meal, vegetarian baked beans, chili beans and refried beans are available in the canned foods section of most supermarkets.

Recently a few companies have introduced precooked, dehydrated beans. These cook in about five minutes. Pinto beans, black beans, split peas, and lentils are some of the varieties that are available. Check your local natural food store for these.

Note the following tips for cooking dried beans.

- Sort through the beans, discard any debris, then rinse thoroughly.
- Soaking beans before cooking reduces their cooking time and increases their digestibility. Soak at least four hours, then pour off soak water and add fresh water for cooking.
- Cook in a large pot with plenty of water. Cover the pot loosely. Use medium-low heat to maintain a low simmer. Check occasionally, adding more water if needed.
- A Crock-Pot is an ideal place to cook beans. The slow, even heat ensures thorough cooking. Start with boiling water and use the highest setting for quickest cooking. For slower cooking, start with cold water and use the highest setting.
- Beans can be cooked very quickly in a pressure cooker. Follow the instructions that came with the cooker.
- Beans should be thoroughly cooked. They should smash easily when pressed between thumb and forefinger.
- Salt toughens the skins of beans and increases the cooking time. It should not be added until the beans are tender.
- Cooked beans may be frozen in airtight containers for later use.

Cutting Fat

Foods that are high in fat are also high in calories. In addition to contributing to unwanted weight gain, a high-fat diet increases your risk for heart disease, adult-onset diabetes, and several forms of cancer. By switching to a plant-based diet you will reduce your intake of fat considerably. The following tips will help you reduce your fat intake even further.

- Choose cooking techniques that do not employ added fat. Baking, grilling, and oven roasting are great alternatives to frying.
- Another fat-cutting cooking trick is to sauté in a liquid such as water or vegetable broth whenever possible. Heat about 1/2

cup of water in a skillet (preferably nonstick) and add the vegetables to be sautéed. Cook over high heat, stirring frequently, until the vegetables are tender. This will take about five minutes. Add a bit more water if necessary to prevent sticking.

- Add onions and garlic to soups and stews at the beginning of the cooking time so their flavors will mellow without sautéing.
- When oil is absolutely necessary to prevent sticking, lightly apply a vegetable oil spray. Another alternative is to start with a very small amount of oil (1 to 2 teaspoons), then add water or vegetable broth as needed to keep the food from sticking.

COOKING DRIED BEANS AND PEAS

BEANS (1 CUP DRY)	AMOUNT OF WATER	COOKING TIME	YIELD
Adzuki beans	3 cups	1½ hours	2¼ cups
Black beans	3 cups	1½ hours	2¼ cups
Black-eyed peas	3 cups	1 hour	2 cups
Chickpeas (garbanzos)	4 cups	2–3 hours	2½ cups
Great Northern beans	3½ cups	2 hours	2 cups
Kidney beans	3 cups	2 hours	2 cups
Lentils	3 cups	1 hour	2¼ cups
Lima beans	2 cups	1½ hours	1½ cups
Navy beans	3 cups	2 hours	2 cups
Pinto beans	3 cups	2½ hours	2¼ cups
Red beans	3 cups	3 hours	2 cups
Soybeans	4 cups	3 hours	2½ cups
Split peas	3 cups	1 hour	2½ cups

- Nonstick pots and pans allow foods to be prepared with little or no fat.
- Choose fat-free dressings for salads. In addition to commercially prepared dressings, seasoned rice vinegar makes a tasty fat-free dressing straight out of the bottle.
- Avoid deep-fried foods and fat-laden pastries. Check your market for low-fat and no-fat alternatives.
- Replace the oil in salad dressing recipes with seasoned rice vinegar, vegetable broth, bean cooking liquid, or water. For a thicker dressing, whisk in a small amount of potato flour.
- Sesame Seasoning (see page 191) is low in fat and delicious on grains, potatoes, and steamed vegetables. Fat-free salad dressing also may be used as a topping for cooked vegetables.
- Applesauce, mashed banana, prune purée, or canned pumpkin may be substituted for all or part of the fat in many baked goods.

Quick Meal and Snack Ideas

- Fresh soybeans (edamame) make a delicious snack or meal addition. You can find them in the freezer section in the supermarket. Cook according to package directions.
- For an instant green salad use pre-washed salad mix and commercially prepared fat-free dressing. Add some canned kidney beans or garbanzo beans for a more substantial meal.
- Baby carrots make a convenient, healthy snack. Try them plain or with Quick Bean Dip (see page 193) or ready-prepared hummus.
- Ramen soup is quick and satisfying. Add some chopped, fresh vegetables for an easy Fast Lane Chow Mein (see page 202).
- Keep a selection of vegetarian soup cups on hand. These are great for quick meals, especially when you're traveling.
- Burritos are quick to make and very portable. They can be eaten hot or cold. For a simple burrito, spread fat-free refried beans on a flour tortilla, add prewashed salad mix and salsa, and roll it up.

- Mix fat-free refried beans with an equal amount of salsa for a delicious bean dip. Serve with baked tortilla chips or fresh vegetables.
- Pita Pizzas (see page 182) are quick and easy to make. Serve them with fat-free Three Bean Salad (commercially prepared, or see page 185).
- A wide variety of fat-free vegetarian cold cuts are available in many supermarkets and natural food stores. These make quick and easy sandwiches.
- Rice cakes and popcorn cakes make great snack foods. Spread them with Quick Bean Dip (see page 193), apple butter, or spreadable fruit.
- Drain garbanzo beans and spoon onto a piece of pita bread. Top with prewashed salad mix and fat-free salad dressing for a quick pocket sandwich.
- Heat a fat-free vegetarian burger patty in the toaster oven. Serve it on a whole grain bun with mustard, ketchup or barbecue sauce, and lettuce. Add sliced red onion and tomato if desired.
- Keep baked or steamed potatoes in the refrigerator. For a quick meal, heat a potato in the microwave and top it with fat-free vegetarian chili and salsa or with Broccoli with Golden Sunshine Sauce (see page 211).
- Arrange chunks of fresh fruit on skewers for quick fruit kabobs.
- Frozen grapes make a refreshing summer snack. To prepare, remove them from the stems and freeze, loosely packed, in an airtight container.
- Frozen bananas make cool snacks or creamy desserts. Peel the bananas, break into chunks, and freeze in airtight containers.

17

Menus for a Week

DAY 1

Breakfast

    Multigrain Cereal (page 175) with raisins

    fortified soy milk or rice milk

    fresh fruit

Lunch

    Pita Pizzas (page 182

    Three Bean Salad (page 185)

    fresh fruit

Dinner

    Neat Loaf (page 206)

    Mashed Potatoes (page 215) and Brown Gravy (page 192)

    Golden Nuggets (page 216)

    Oatmeal Cookies (page 223)

Day 2

Breakfast

French Toast (page 173)

Corn Butter (page 191)

maple syrup or spreadable fruit

fresh fruit

Lunch

Burritos Supreme (page 181)

Rainbow Salad (page 186)

Strawberry Smoothie (page 226)

Dinner

Spaghetti (page 203)

Broccoli with Golden Sunshine Sauce (page 211)

Garlic Bread (page 218)

Chocolate Pudding (page 224)

Day 3

Breakfast

Whole Wheat Pancakes (page 172)

Corn Butter (page 191)

maple syrup or spreadable fruit

fresh fruit

Lunch

Split Pea Soup (page 196)

whole grain bread or roll

Potato Salad (page 186)

Dinner

Very Primo Pasta (page 200)

Desi's Carrot Coins (page 188)

green salad with Simple Vinaigrette (page 188)

Fruit Gel (page 224)

DAY 4

Breakfast

   Oatmeal Waffles (page 173)

   Corn Butter (page 191)

   fresh fruit or spreadable fruit

Lunch

   Missing Egg Sandwich (page 180)

   Alphabet Soup (page 196)

   fresh fruit

Dinner

   Terrific Tacos (page 201)

   Oven Fries (page 213)

   carrot sticks

   Orange Power Pops (page 225)

DAY 5

Breakfast

   Pumpkin Spice Muffins (page 219

   cold cereal

   fortified soy milk or rice milk

   fresh fruit

Lunch

   Beanie Weenies (page 205)

   green salad with Creamy Dill Dressing (page 189)

   watermelon

Dinner

   Fast Lane Chow Mein (page 202)

   Sesame Asparagus (page 213)

   Winter Squash with Peanut Sauce (page 217)

   Nutty Fruitballs (page 225)

Day 6

Breakfast

    Scrambled Tofu (page 174)

    whole grain toast with Corn Butter (page 191)

    Strawberry Sauce (page 195) or spreadable fruit

Lunch

    Broccoli Potato Soup (page 199)

    Neat Loaf sandwich (page 206)

    whole grain bread

Dinner

    Baked Beans (page 208)

    Rainbow Salad (leftover from Day 3)

    Quick and Easy Brown Bread (page 219)

Day 7

Breakfast

    Maple Walnut Granola (page 175)

    fortified soy milk or rice milk

    fresh fruit

Lunch

    Quickie Quesadillas (page 181)

    Quick Chili Beans (page 209)

    green salad

Dinner

    Barbecue-style Baked Tofu (page 208)

    Brown Rice (page 176)

    Crispy Green Salad (page 187)

    Apple Crisp (page 221)

18

The Recipes

BREAKFASTS

Whole Wheat Pancakes
MAKES 24 2-INCH PANCAKES

Six simple ingredients are all it takes to make these nutritious whole-grain pancakes. They are delicious with fresh fruit, unsweetened spreadable fruit (see Glossary), or maple syrup.

1 banana
1¼ cups fortified soy milk or rice milk
1 tablespoon maple syrup
1 cup whole wheat pastry flour or whole wheat flour

2 teaspoons sodium-free baking powder
¼ teaspoon salt
vegetable oil cooking spray

Mash banana in a large bowl, then stir in milk and maple syrup.

In a separate bowl mix flour, baking powder, and salt. Add to banana mixture and stir until smooth.

Pour small amounts of batter onto a preheated nonstick, lightly oil-sprayed griddle or skillet and cook until tops bubble. Flip with a spatula and cook second side until golden brown, about 1 minute. Serve immediately.

Per pancake: 42 calories; 2 g protein; 9 g carbohydrate;
0.5 g fat; 1 g fiber; 37 mg sodium; calories from protein: 14%;
calories from carbohydrates: 75%; calories from fats: 11%

• • •

Oatmeal Waffles

MAKES 6 WAFFLES

These easily prepared waffles are a delicious way to add healthful oats to your diet.

2 cups rolled oats	1 teaspoon vanilla
2 cups water	vegetable oil cooking spray
1 banana	fresh fruit, spreadable fruit, or
¼ teaspoon salt	maple syrup for serving
1 tablespoon maple syrup	

Preheat waffle iron to medium-high.

Combine oats, water, banana, salt, maple syrup, and vanilla in a blender. Blend on high speed until completely smooth.

Lightly spray waffle iron with cooking spray. Pour in enough batter to just barely reach edges and cook until golden brown, 5 to 10 minutes. without lifting lid.

Note: The batter should be pourable. If it becomes too thick as it stands, add a bit more water to achieve desired consistency.

Serve with fresh fruit, spreadable fruit, or syrup.

Per waffle: 130 calories; 5 g protein; 25 g carbohydrate; 2 g fat; 3 g fiber;
90 mg sodium; calories from protein: 14%;
calories from carbohydrates: 74%; calories from fats: 12%

• • •

French Toast

MAKES 6 SLICES

This cholesterol-free French toast tastes great as it adds beneficial soy and whole wheat to your diet.

1 cup fortified soy milk (plain or vanilla)	1 teaspoon vanilla
¼ cup whole wheat pastry flour	½ teaspoon cinnamon
1 tablespoon maple syrup	6 slices whole grain bread
	vegetable oil cooking spray

Combine milk, flour, maple syrup, vanilla, and cinnamon in a blender. Blend until smooth, then pour into a flat dish.

Soak bread slices in batter until soft but not soggy. The amount of time this takes will vary depending on the bread used.

Cook in an oil-sprayed nonstick skillet over medium heat until first side is golden brown, about 3 minutes. Turn carefully with a spatula and cook second side until brown, about 3 minutes.

Per slice: 129 calories; 6 g protein; 23 g carbohydrate; 2 g fat;
4 g fiber; 191 mg sodium; calories from protein: 17%;
calories from carbohydrates: 68%; calories from fats: 15%

• • •

Scrambled Tofu

MAKES 2 ½-CUP SERVINGS

This nutritious golden scramble is especially good with toasted English muffins. You can also wrap it in a whole wheat tortilla for a delicious breakfast burrito.

2 teaspoons toasted sesame oil
¼ cup finely chopped onion
½ pound firm tofu, crumbled
¼ teaspoon garlic granules

¼ teaspoon turmeric
¼ teaspoon cumin
⅛ teaspoon black pepper
2 teaspoons soy sauce

Heat oil in a nonstick skillet. Add onion and cook over medium heat, stirring often, for 3 minutes. Add tofu, garlic granules, turmeric, cumin, black pepper, and soy sauce. Cook, stirring gently for 3 to 5 minutes.

Per ½-cup serving: 137 calories; 10 g protein; 4 g carbohydrate;
10 g fat; 2 g fiber; 177 mg sodium; calories from protein: 27%;
calories from carbohydrates: 11%; calories from fats: 62%

• • •

Quick Breakfast Pudding

MAKES 4 1-CUP SERVINGS

Dried fruit and oatmeal make a sweet, creamy breakfast cereal.

8 dried apricot halves
5 or 6 dried figs
¼ cup raisins
1 green apple (Pippin or Granny Smith)

1 cup quick rolled oats
3 cups fortified vanilla soy milk or rice milk
½ teaspoon cinnamon

Chop apricots, figs, and raisins in a food processor.

Cut apple in quarters and remove core. Add to dried fruit in food processor and chop fine.

Transfer to a saucepan and add oats, milk, and cinnamon. Heat to a simmer, then cover and cook, stirring occasionally, until thickened, about 5 minutes.

Per 1-cup serving: 272 calories; 10 g protein; 52 g carbohydrate;
6 g fat; 8 g fiber; 26 mg sodium; calories from protein: 13%;
calories from carbohydrates: 71%; calories from fats: 16%

• • •

Maple Walnut Granola
MAKES ABOUT 6 CUPS (12 ½-CUP SERVINGS)

This yummy granola is made without added oil.

3 cups rolled oats	¼ cup sesame seeds
1 cup wheat germ	¼ cup maple syrup
½ cup chopped walnuts	2 tablespoons molasses
½ cup raisins	1 teaspoon cinnamon
½ cup dried cranberries (optional)	

Preheat oven to 300°F.

Combine all ingredients in a large bowl and mix thoroughly.

Transfer to a 9-by-13-inch baking dish. Bake, turning often with a spatula, until mixture is golden brown, about 25 minutes. Store in an airtight container.

Per ½-cup serving: 202 calories; 7 g protein; 31 g carbohydrate;
7 g fat; 4 g fiber; 5 mg sodium; calories from protein: 12%;
calories from carbohydrates: 59%; calories from fats: 29%

• • •

Multigrain Cereal
MAKES 2½ 1-CUP SERVINGS

Multigrain hot cereals provide great flavor as well as the nutritional benefits of several whole grains. A variety of multigrain cereal mixes are available in natural food stores and many supermarkets. One of the most delicious and most widely distributed is Bob's Red Mill 10 Grain Cereal (see Glossary). Use this method for cooking any of these hearty, satisfying breakfast cereals.

1 cup multigrain cereal mix	3 cups boiling water
½ teaspoon salt (optional)	

Stir cereal and salt into boiling water in a saucepan. Cover loosely and simmer, stirring occasionally, for 7 minutes.

Remove from heat and let stand, covered, for 10 minutes before serving.

Health hint: By gradually reducing the amount of salt you add, you can re-educate your taste buds so that the cereal will taste fine with no salt at all.

> Per 1-cup serving: 200 calories; 6 g protein; 40 g carbohydrate;
> 2 g fat; 4 g fiber; 10 to 580 mg sodium (depending on amount
> of salt used in recipe); calories from protein: 13%;
> calories from carbohydrates: 77%; calories from fats: 10%

● ● ●

GRAINS AND PASTAS

Brown Rice

MAKES 3 1-CUP SERVINGS

Flavorful and satisfying, brown rice is an excellent source of protective soluble fiber. In the cooking method described below, the rice is toasted, then simmered in plenty of water (like pasta) to enhance its flavor and reduce cooking time.

1 cup short- or long-grain brown rice	4 cups boiling water
	½ teaspoon salt

Rinse rice in cool water. Drain off as much water as possible. Place rice in a saucepan over medium heat, stirring constantly until completely dry, 3 to 5 minutes.

Add boiling water and salt, then cover and simmer until rice is just tender, about 35 minutes. Pour off excess liquid (this can be saved and used as a broth for soups and stews if desired).

> Per 1-cup serving: 228 calories; 5 g protein; 48 g carbohydrate;
> 2 g fat; 2 g fiber; 360 mg sodium; calories from protein: 9%;
> calories from carbohydrates: 84%; calories from fats: 7%

● ● ●

Brown Rice and Barley

MAKES ABOUT 6 1-CUP SERVINGS

The addition of whole barley adds great texture to brown rice. Hulled barley, which is a bit less refined and slightly more nutritious than pearled barley, is sold in many natural food stores.

1   cup short-grain brown rice   1   teaspoon salt
1   cup hulled or pearled barley

Bring 4 cups water to a boil; add rice, barley, and salt. Reduce heat to a simmer, then cover and cook until grains are tender and all the water is absorbed, about 45 minutes.

> Per 1-cup serving: 222 calories; 6 g protein; 46 g carbohydrate;
> 2 g fat; 6 g fiber; 362 mg sodium; calories from protein: 11%;
> calories from carbohydrates: 81%; calories from fats: 8%

● ● ●

Quick Confetti Rice
MAKES 3 1-CUP SERVINGS

This colorful rice pilaf is made with no added fat, so be sure to use a nonstick skillet.

2   tablespoons water or Vegetable Broth (page 195)
2   cups cooked Brown Rice (page 176)
½ cup frozen corn

½ cup frozen peas
½ red bell pepper, diced
½ teaspoon curry powder
¼ cup golden raisins (optional)

Heat water in a large nonstick skillet. Add cooked rice, then use a spatula or the back of a wooden spoon to separate kernels.

Add corn, peas, bell pepper, curry powder, and raisins. Cook over medium heat, stirring often, until very hot, about 5 minutes.

> Per 1-cup serving: 232 calories; 6 g protein; 52 g carbohydrate;
> 1.2 g fat; 6 g fiber; 210 mg sodium (if rice is cooked with salt);
> calories from protein: 10%; calories from carbohydrates: 85%;
> calories from fats: 5%

● ● ●

Bulgur
MAKES 2½ CUPS (2 1-CUP SERVINGS)

Bulgur is made from whole wheat kernels that have been cracked and toasted, giving it a delicious, nutty flavor. It cooks quickly and may be served plain, or in a pilaf or salad. It is sold in natural food stores, and in some supermarkets, usually in the bulk food section.

1   cup uncooked bulgur   2   cups boiling water
½ teaspoon salt

Mix bulgur and salt in a large bowl. Stir in boiling water. Cover and let stand until tender, about 25 minutes.

Alternate cooking method: Stir bulgur and salt into boiling water in a saucepan. Reduce heat to a simmer, then cover and cook without stirring until bulgur is tender, about 15 minutes.

> Per 1-cup serving: 192 calories; 6 g protein; 42 g carbohydrate;
> 0.8 g fat; 10 g fiber; 436 mg sodium; calories from protein: 13%;
> calories from carbohydrates: 84%; calories from fats: 3%

● ● ●

Whole Wheat Couscous
MAKES 3 1-CUP SERVINGS

Couscous is actually pasta that takes only minutes to prepare. It makes a delicious side dish or salad base. Whole wheat couscous, which contains fiber and more vitamins and minerals than refined couscous, is sold in natural food stores and some supermarkets.

1 cup whole wheat couscous   1½ cups boiling water
½ teaspoon salt

Stir couscous and salt into boiling water in a saucepan. Remove from heat and cover. Let stand 10 to 15 minutes, then fluff with a fork and serve.

> Per 1-cup serving: 200 calories; 6 g protein; 42 g carbohydrate;
> 0.2 g fat; 4 g fiber; 364 mg sodium; calories from protein: 14%;
> calories from carbohydrates: 85%; calories from fats: 1%

● ● ●

Polenta
MAKES 4 1-CUP SERVINGS

Polenta, or coarsely ground cornmeal, is easy to prepare and tremendously versatile. When it is first cooked it is soft, like Cream of Wheat, and perfect for breakfast topped with fruit and fortified soy milk, or for dinner topped with vegetables and a savory sauce. When chilled, it becomes firm and sliceable, perfect for grilling or sautéing.

5 cups water   1 teaspoon thyme (optional)
1 cup polenta   1 teaspoon oregano (optional)
1 teaspoon salt

Measure water into a large pot, then whisk in polenta, salt, and herbs, if using.

Simmer over medium heat, stirring often, until very thick, about 25 minutes.

Serve hot or transfer to a 9-by-13-inch baking dish and chill until firm.

For grilled polenta, turn cold polenta out of the pan onto a cutting board and cut it with a sharp knife into ½-inch-thick slices. Lightly spray a large nonstick skillet with vegetable oil cooking spray and place it over medium-high heat. Arrange polenta slices in a single layer about 1 inch apart and cook 5 minutes. Turn and cook second side 5 minutes. Repeat with remaining polenta.

> Per 1-cup serving: 110 calories; 2 g protein; 23 g carbohydrate;
> 2 g fiber; 1 g fat; 592 mg sodium; calories from protein: 9%;
> calories from carbohydrates: 82%; calories from fats: 9%

● ● ●

Quinoa
MAKES 3 1-CUP SERVINGS

Quinoa ("keen-wah") comes from the high plains of the Andes Mountains, where it is nicknamed "the mother grain" for its life-giving properties. The National Academy of Sciences has called quinoa "one of the best sources of protein in the vegetable kingdom," because of its excellent amino acid pattern. Quinoa cooks quickly, and as it cooks the germ unfolds like a little tail. It has a light, fluffy texture, and may be eaten plain, used as a pilaf, or as an addition to soups and stews. The dry grain is coated with a bitter-tasting substance called saponin, which repels insects and birds and protects it from ultraviolet radiation. Quinoa must be washed thoroughly before cooking to remove this bitter coating. The easiest way to wash it is to place it in a strainer and rinse it with cool water until the water runs clear.

1   cup quinoa   2   cups boiling water

Rinse quinoa thoroughly in a fine sieve, then add it to boiling water in a saucepan. Reduce to a simmer, then cover loosely and cook until quinoa is tender and fluffy, about 15 minutes.

> Per 1-cup serving: 212 calories; 8 g protein; 40 g carbohydrate;
> 4 g fat; 4 g fiber; 12 mg sodium; calories from protein: 14%;
> calories from carbohydrates: 72%; calories from fats: 14%

● ● ●

SANDWICHES AND WRAPS

Missing Egg Sandwich
MAKES 6 SANDWICHES

These sandwiches have the flavor and appearance of egg salad without the saturated fat and cholesterol.

½ pound firm reduced-fat tofu (1 cup)
1 green onion, finely chopped, including green top
2 tablespoons pickle relish
2 tablespoons Tofu Mayo (page 190) or vegan mayonnaise
2 teaspoons stone-ground mustard
2 teaspoons reduced-sodium soy sauce
¼ teaspoon cumin
¼ teaspoon turmeric
¼ teaspoon garlic powder
12 slices whole grain bread
6 lettuce leaves
6 tomato slices

Mash tofu, leaving some chunks. Add green onion, pickle relish, Tofu Mayo, mustard, soy sauce, cumin, turmeric, and garlic powder. Mix well.

Spread on 6 slices of bread. Garnish with lettuce and tomato slices, and top with remaining bread.

Per sandwich: 246 calories; 15 g protein; 38 g carbohydrate; 6 g fat; 6 g fiber; 452 mg sodium; calories from protein: 20%; calories from carbohydrates: 58%; calories from fats: 22%

● ● ●

Banana and Raisin Sandwich
MAKES 2 SANDWICHES

Children love this sweet filling combination. This sandwich would be great for breakfast, lunch, or snack.

4 tablespoons natural peanut butter
4 slices whole grain bread
1 banana, sliced
2 or 3 tablespoons raisins

Spread peanut butter evenly on 2 slices of bread. Top with sliced banana and sprinkle with raisins. Top with remaining bread.

Per ½ sandwich: 203 calories; 7 g protein; 27 g carbohydrate; 9 g fat; 4 g fiber; 124 mg sodium; calories from protein: 13%; calories from carbohydrates: 50%; calories from fats: 37%

● ● ●

Burritos Supremos

MAKES 4 BURRITOS

Wrap up rice and beans for a meal to enjoy at home or on the go.

1   15-ounce can vegetarian refried beans
4   flour tortillas
1   cup cooked Brown Rice (page 176) (optional)
1   cup shredded romaine lettuce

1   tomato, diced
2   green onions, sliced
½ avocado, peeled and sliced (optional)
½ cup salsa

Heat beans in a saucepan or microwave.

Warm tortillas, one at a time, in a large dry skillet, flipping to warm both sides until soft and pliable.

Spread warm tortilla with approximately ½ cup of the beans and ¼ cup rice if using.

Top with lettuce, tomato, onions, avocado if using, and salsa. Roll tortilla around filling.

Serve or wrap in plastic and refrigerate.

Per burrito: 310 calories; 12 g protein; 51 g carbohydrate;
8 g fat; 8 g fiber; 732 mg sodium; calories from protein: 15%;
calories from carbohydrates: 64%; calories from fats: 21%

● ● ●

Quickie Quesadillas

MAKES 8 SERVINGS

These quesadillas are a truly happy marriage between cultures: Middle Eastern red pepper hummus served with Mexican corn tortillas and garnished with salsa makes an absolutely delicious meal or snack.

1   15-ounce can garbanzo beans
½ cup water-packed roasted red pepper
3   tablespoons lemon juice
1   tablespoon tahini (sesame butter)

1   garlic clove, peeled
¼ teaspoon cumin
8   corn tortillas
½ cup chopped green onions
½ cup tomatoes, diced
½ to 1 cup salsa

Drain garbanzo beans and place in a food processor or blender with roasted peppers, lemon juice, tahini, garlic, and cumin. Process until very smooth, 1 to 2 minutes.

Spread a tortilla with 2 to 3 tablespoons of garbanzo mixture and place in a large nonstick skillet over medium heat. Sprinkle with chopped green onions, diced tomatoes, and salsa.

Top with a second tortilla and cook until bottom tortilla is warm and soft, 2 to 3 minutes. Turn and cook second side for another minute. Remove from pan and cut in half. Repeat with remaining tortillas.

Per ½ quesadilla: 129 calories; 5 g protein; 22 g carbohydrate;
3 g fat; 2 g fiber; 160 mg sodium; calories from protein: 15%;
calories from carbohydrates: 67%; calories from fats: 18%

● ● ●

Pita Pizzas

MAKES 6 PIZZAS

Whole wheat pita bread makes a perfect crust for a child-size pizza, and children enjoy assembling them once the vegetables have been chopped. In addition to the toppings listed, you could also add fat-free vegetarian pepperoni slices. Yves Veggie Pepperoni and Smart Deli Thin Slices by Lightlife are two delicious options.

1   15-ounce can tomato sauce
1   6-ounce can tomato paste
1   teaspoon garlic granules or powder
½ teaspoon dried basil
½ teaspoon dried oregano

½ teaspoon dried thyme
6   pieces whole wheat pita bread
2   green onions, thinly sliced
1   red bell pepper, diced
1   cup chopped mushrooms

Preheat oven to 375°F.

Combine tomato sauce, tomato paste, garlic granules, and herbs.

Turn a piece of pita bread upside down and spread with 2 to 3 table-spoons of sauce. Top with chopped vegetables. Repeat with remaining pita breads. Arrange on a baking sheet and bake until edges are lightly browned, about 10 minutes.

Note: You will only use about half the sauce. Refrigerate or freeze the remainder for use at another time.

Per pizza: 153 calories; 6 g protein; 32 g carbohydrate; 1 g fat;
5 g fiber; 567 mg sodium; calories from protein: 14%;
calories from carbohydrates: 78%; calories from fats: 8%

Meatlike Sandwiches, Burgers, and Hot Dogs

A wide variety of meatless cold cuts, burgers, and hot dogs are sold in natural food stores and most supermarkets. A sampling of these products is shown below. Check the deli case as well as the freezer section for these products and others. Be sure to read the ingredient list to determine that there are no animal ingredients, such as eggs, egg whites, cheese, whey, or casein. Check the nutritional information as well to determine the amounts of fat and sodium.

MEATLESS COLD CUTS AND DELI SLICES

Smart Bacon (Lightlife Foods)

Foney Baloney (Lightlife Foods)

Smart Deli Turkey (Lightlife Foods)

Smart Deli Bologna (Lightlife Foods)

Smart Deli Ham (Lightlife Foods)

Soylami (Lightlife Foods)

Pepperoni (Lightlife Foods)

Lean Links Sausage (Lightlife Foods)

Veggie Bologna Slices (Yves Fine Foods)

Veggie Pizza Pepperoni Slices (Yves Fine Foods)

Veggie Ham Slices (Yves Fine Foods)

Veggie Turkey Slices (Yves Fine Foods)

Veggie Salami Slices (Yves Fine Foods)

MEATLESS BURGERS

Veggie Cuisine Burger (Yves Fine Foods)

Veggie Burger Burgers (Yves Fine Foods)

Garden Vegetable Patties (Yves Fine Foods)

Black Bean and Mushroom Burgers (Yves Fine Foods)

Veggie Chick'n Burger (Yves Fine Foods)

LightBurgers (Lightlife Foods)

Prime Burger (White Wave Inc.)

Green Giant Harvest Burger (Pillsbury Company)
Vegan Original Boca Burger (Boca Burger Company)
Superburgers (Turtle Island Foods)
Natural Touch Vegan Burger (Worthington Foods)
Garden Vegan Burger (Wholesome and Hearty Foods)
Gardenburger Hamburger Style (Wholesome and Hearty Foods)
Amy's California Veggie Burger (Amy's Kitchen)
Amy's All American Burger (Amy's Kitchen)
Soy Deli All Natural Tofu Burger (Qwong Hop & Company)

MEATLESS HOT DOGS

Veggie Dogs (Yves Fine Foods)
Jumbo Veggie Dogs (Yves Fine Foods)
Hot & Spicy Jumbo Veggie Dogs
Good Dogs (Yves Fine Foods)
Tofu Dogs (Yves Fine Foods)
Smart Dogs (Lightlife Foods)
Wild Dogs (Wildwood Natural Foods)

OTHER MEATLESS PRODUCTS

Smart Ground (Lightlife Foods)
Veggie Ground Round Original (Yves Fine Foods)
Veggie Ground Round Italian (Yves Fine Foods)
Veggie Breakfast Links (Yves Fine Foods)
Canadian Veggie Bacon (Yves Fine Foods)
Veggie Breakfast Patties (Yves Fine Foods)
Chiken Chunks (Harvest Direct)
Chiken Breasts (Harvest Direct)
Tofurky Deli Slices (Turtle Island Foods)
Tofurky Jerky (Turtle Island Foods)
Not Chicken Deli Slices (United Specialty Foods)
White Wave Sandwich Slices (White Wave Foods)

SALADS

Three Bean Salad

MAKES 6 1-CUP SERVINGS

This traditional salad is quick to make and keeps well. For a quick meal, serve it on a bed of romaine lettuce leaves with a slice or two of whole grain bread.

1   15-ounce can kidney beans, drained
1   15-ounce can garbanzo beans, drained
1   15-ounce can green beans, drained
¼ cup finely chopped red onion
¼ cup finely chopped fresh parsley

½ cup cider vinegar
¼ cup seasoned rice vinegar
3   garlic cloves, pressed or minced
2   tablespoons chopped fresh basil or ½ teaspoon dried basil
½ teaspoon dried oregano
½ teaspoon dried marjoram
¼ teaspoon black pepper

Place drained beans in a large bowl with chopped onion and parsley. Stir together vinegars, garlic, herbs, and pepper. Add to beans and toss to mix. Chill 2 to 3 hours before serving if time permits.

Per 1-cup serving: 180 calories; 10 g protein; 34 g carbohydrate; 2 g fat; 10 g fiber; 360 mg sodium; calories from protein: 21%; calories from carbohydrates: 72%; calories from fats: 7%

● ● ●

California Waldorf Salad

MAKES ABOUT 6 1-CUP SERVINGS

2   crisp, tangy apples (Fuji, winesap, Granny Smith, or similar)
1   large carrot, julienned or grated
½ cup raisins
¼ cup chopped walnuts

⅓ cup Tofu Mayo (page 190) or vegan mayonnaise
3   tablespoons seasoned rice vinegar

Scrub and dice apples, then place into a salad bowl. Add carrots, raisins, and walnuts. Mix Tofu Mayo and vinegar. Add to salad and stir to mix. Chill before serving if possible.

Per 1-cup serving: 122 calories; 2 g protein; 22 g carbohydrate; 4 g fat; 2 g fiber; 306 mg sodium; calories from protein: 7%; calories from carbohydrates: 67%; calories from fats: 26%

● ● ●

Potato Salad

MAKES 5 1-CUP SERVINGS

This delicious, creamy potato salad contains no cholesterol and is surprisingly low in fat.

4 medium potatoes, diced
2 celery stalks, thinly sliced, including leaves
3 green onions, chopped
¼ cup finely chopped fresh parsley
3 tablespoons seasoned rice vinegar

⅓ cup Tofu Mayo (page 190) or vegan mayonnaise
1½ tablespoons stone-ground mustard
¼ to ½ teaspoon salt
⅛ teaspoon black pepper

Steam potatoes over boiling water until just barely tender, about 15 minutes, then transfer to a large bowl.

Add celery, onions, parsley, and vinegar. Stir to mix.

Stir in Tofu Mayo, mustard, salt, and pepper and toss gently. Chill before serving, if time allows.

Per 1-cup serving: 204 calories; 6 g protein; 50 g carbohydrate;
1 g fat; 4 g fiber; 428-534 mg sodium; calories from protein: 10%;
calories from carbohydrates: 86%; calories from fats: 4%

● ● ●

Rainbow Salad

MAKES 12 ½-CUP SERVINGS

Cabbage and carrots team up to make a beautiful and delicious salad.

2 cups shredded green cabbage
2 cups shredded purple cabbage
2 carrots, grated or julienned
2 celery stalks, thinly sliced
3 green onions, sliced
1 apple, finely chopped or julienned

1 tablespoon lemon juice
½ cup Tofu Mayo (page 190) or vegan mayonnaise
⅓ cup apple juice concentrate

Combine cabbage, carrots, celery, and green onions in a salad bowl. Toss apple with lemon juice and add to salad. Add Tofu Mayo and apple juice concentrate and mix well. If possible, chill before serving.

Per ½-cup serving: 40 calories; 1 g protein; 9 g carbohydrate;
0.1 g fat; 1 g fiber; 87 mg sodium; calories from protein: 7%;
calories from carbohydrates: 89%; calories from fats: 4%

● ● ●

Chinese Noodle Salad

MAKES 10 1-CUP SERVINGS

This vegetarian version of Chinese Chicken Salad is always a hit. It is easy to make and keeps well, so it can be enjoyed for several meals. The noodles in the salad come from a package of ramen soup mix, available in natural food stores and many supermarkets. The seasoning packet is used to make the dressing. Be sure to select a variety in which the noodles are baked instead of fried, and be sure the seasonings do not contain meat or other animal products. Two vegetarian brands are Westbrae and Soken.

1 medium head green cabbage, finely shredded (about 8 cups)
½ cup slivered almonds
¼ cup sesame seeds
3 or 4 green onions, thinly sliced or ½ cup finely chopped red onion
1 package vegetarian ramen soup, any flavor

1 tablespoon toasted sesame oil
⅓ cup seasoned rice vinegar
2 tablespoons sugar or other sweetener
½ teaspoon black pepper
fresh cilantro (optional)

Preheat oven to 375°F.

Place shredded cabbage in a large salad bowl.

Toast almonds and sesame seeds in an ovenproof dish in oven (or toaster oven) for 8 to 10 minutes, until lightly browned and fragrant. Add to shredded cabbage, along with the onions. Coarsely crush uncooked ramen noodles and add them to the salad.

Empty the packet of seasoning mix into a small bowl or jar, then stir in toasted sesame oil, seasoned rice vinegar, sugar, and pepper. Mix thoroughly and pour over the salad. Toss to mix, and then allow to stand 30 minutes in order for the noodles to soften. Garnish with fresh cilantro just before serving, if desired.

Per 1-cup serving: 144 calories; 8 g protein; 26 g carbohydrate;
2 g fat; 8 g fiber; 450 mg sodium; calories from protein: 22%;
calories from carbohydrates: 69%; calories from fats: 9%

● ● ●

Crispy Green Salad

MAKES 10 1-CUP SERVINGS

Tahini, or sesame seed butter; miso made from fermented soybeans; and toasted sesame oil give this salad its unique flavor and aroma. You can find these ingredients in large supermarkets or international groceries.

8 cups torn romaine lettuce
2 cups finely shredded green cabbage
1 cup thinly sliced celery (about 2 stalks)
1 tablespoon tahini
1 tablespoon seasoned rice vinegar

1½ teaspoons white miso
1 teaspoon toasted sesame oil
½ teaspoon sugar
1 small garlic clove, pressed or minced
1 or 2 tablespoons water

Mix lettuce, cabbage, and celery in a salad bowl.

In a small bowl combine tahini, vinegar, miso, oil, sugar, and garlic. Blend until smooth, adding enough water to produce a thick but pourable consistency.

Just before serving, pour dressing over salad and toss to mix.

Per 1-cup serving: 31 calories; 1 g protein; 4 g carbohydrate;
1.5 g fat; 1 g fiber; 101 mg sodium; calories from protein: 17%;
calories from carbohydrates: 43%; calories from fats: 40%

● ● ●

Desi's Carrot Coins
MAKES ABOUT 2 1-CUP SERVINGS

Desi, a 9-year-old budding chef, shows us how delicious fresh vegetables are with just a bit of lemon (or lime) juice and salt. These are great for snacking or added to other salads.

2 carrots
2 tablespoons lemon or lime juice

¼ teaspoon salt

Cut carrots into ¼-inch-thick rounds (coins) and place them in a bowl. Sprinkle with lemon or lime juice and salt. Let stand 20 minutes before serving.

Per 1-cup serving: 34 calories; 0.8 g protein; 8 g carbohydrate;
0.1 g fat; 2 g fiber; 158 mg sodium; calories from protein: 8%;
calories from carbohydrates: 88%; calories from fats: 4%

DIPS, DRESSINGS, AND SAUCES

Simple Vinaigrette
MAKES ½ CUP

Seasoned rice vinegar makes a delicious salad dressing all by itself, or enhanced with mustard and garlic.

½ cup seasoned rice vinegar
1 to 2 teaspoons stone-ground or
  Dijon-style mustard

1   clove garlic, pressed

Whisk all ingredients together. Use as a dressing for salads and for steamed vegetables.

> Per 1 tablespoon: 27 calories; 0.1 g protein; 6 g carbohydrate;
> 0.1 g fat; 0 g fiber; 562 mg sodium; calories from protein: 2%;
> calories from carbohydrates: 94%; calories from fats: 4%

• • •

Balsamic Vinaigrette
MAKES ¼ CUP

The mellow flavor of balsamic vinegar is delicious on salads.

2   tablespoons balsamic vinegar
2   tablespoons seasoned rice
    vinegar

1   tablespoon ketchup
1   teaspoon stone-ground mustard
1   garlic clove, pressed

Whisk vinegars, ketchup, mustard, and garlic together.

> Per 1 tablespoon: 20 calories; 0.1 g protein; 4.5 g carbohydrate;
> 0.08 g fat; 0.05 g fiber; 229 mg sodium; calories from protein: 3%;
> calories from carbohydrates: 93%; calories from fats: 4 %

• • •

Creamy Dill Dressing
MAKES ABOUT 1½ CUPS

This rich-tasting, creamy dressing has no added oil. Its creaminess comes from tofu.

1   12.3-ounce package Mori-Nu
    firm tofu
2   tablespoons lemon juice
3   tablespoons seasoned rice
    vinegar

1   tablespoon cider vinegar
1   teaspoon garlic granules or pow-
    der
½ teaspoon dill weed
¼ teaspoon salt

Combine all ingredients in a food processor or blender. Blend until completely smooth, 1 to 2 minutes. Store any extra dressing in an airtight container in the refrigerator.

> Per 1 tablespoon: 12 calories; 1 g protein; 1 g carbohydrate; 1 g fat;
> 0.1 g fiber; 90 mg sodium; calories from protein: 36%;
> calories from carbohydrates: 18%; calories from fats: 46%

• • •

Tofu Mayo

Makes about 1½ cups

Use this low-fat mayonnaise substitute on sandwiches and salads.

1 12.3-ounce package Mori-Nu
   Lite Silken Tofu (firm or extra
   firm)
¾ teaspoon salt
½ teaspoon sugar

1 teaspoon Dijon mustard
1½ tablespoons lemon juice
1½ tablespoons seasoned rice
   vinegar

Combine tofu, salt, sugar, mustard, lemon juice, and vinegar in a food processor or blender, and process until completely smooth, 1 to 2 minutes. Chill thoroughly before using.

Per 1 tablespoon: 6 calories; 1 g protein; 0.4 g carbohydrate;
0.1 g fat; 0 g fiber; 93 mg sodium; calories from protein: 48%;
calories from carbohydrates: 29%; calories from fats: 23%

• • •

Salsa Fresca

Makes about 6 cups

This fresh and chunky salsa is quite mild. For a hotter salsa, increase the jalapeños or red pepper flakes.

4 large ripe tomatoes, chopped
   (about 4 cups)
1 small onion, finely chopped
1 bell pepper, finely chopped
1 jalapeño pepper, seeded and
   finely chopped or 1 teaspoon red
   pepper flakes

4 garlic cloves, minced
1 cup chopped cilantro leaves
1 15-ounce can tomato sauce
2 tablespoons cider vinegar
1½ teaspoons cumin

Combine all ingredients in a mixing bowl. Stir to mix. Let stand 1 hour before serving.

Note: Salsa will keep in the refrigerator for about 2 weeks. It also freezes well.

Per 1 tablespoon: 4 calories; 0.1 g protein; 1 g carbohydrate;
0.03 g fat; 0.2 g fiber; 27 mg sodium; calories from protein: 14%;
calories from carbohydrates: 79%; calories from fats: 7%

• • •

Sesame Salt
MAKES ½ CUP

Sesame Salt is a delicious alternative to butter or margarine on cooked grains, baked potatoes, or steamed vegetables. Unhulled sesame seeds (sometimes called "brown sesame seeds") are sold in natural food stores and some supermarkets.

½ cup unhulled sesame seeds   ½ teaspoon salt

Toast sesame seeds in a dry skillet over medium heat, stirring constantly until they begin to pop and brown slightly, about 5 minutes. Transfer to a blender. Add salt and grind into a uniform powder. Transfer to an airtight container. Store in refrigerator.

> Per 1 tablespoon: 52 calories; 2 g protein; 2 g carbohydrate;
> 4 g fat; 1 g fiber; 134 mg sodium; calories from protein: 12%;
> calories from carbohydrates: 15%; calories from fats: 73%

● ● ●

Sesame Seasoning
MAKES ½ CUP

Sesame Seasoning is delicious with steamed vegetables, cooked grains, and legumes. Unhulled sesame seeds are light brown in color and are sold in natural food stores and some supermarkets.

½ cup unhulled sesame seeds   2 tablespoons nutritional yeast
½ teaspoon salt

Toast sesame seeds in a dry skillet over medium heat. Stir constantly until seeds begin to pop and brown slightly, about 5 minutes.

Transfer to a blender, add salt and nutritional yeast and grind into a fine powder.

Transfer to an airtight container. Store in refrigerator.

> Per 1 tablespoon: 57 calories; 2 g protein; 3 g carbohydrate;
> 4 g fat; 1 g fiber; 137 mg sodium; calories from protein: 15%;
> calories from carbohydrates: 19%; calories from fats: 66%

● ● ●

Corn Butter
MAKES ABOUT 2 CUPS

This creamy yellow spread is a low-fat alternative to margarine. Emes Jel and agar powder are thickening agents that are sold in natural food stores.

¼ cup cornmeal

2 teaspoons Emes Jel (see Glossary) or 1½ teaspoons agar powder

1 cup boiling water

2 tablespoons raw cashews

½ teaspoon salt

2 teaspoons lemon juice

1 tablespoon finely grated raw carrot

1 teaspoon nutritional yeast (optional)

Combine cornmeal with 1 cup water in a small saucepan. Simmer, stirring frequently, until very thick, about 10 minutes. Set aside.

Combine Emes Jel or agar powder with ¼ cup cold water in a blender. Let stand at least 3 minutes. Add 1 cup boiling water and blend to mix. Add cooked cornmeal, cashews, salt, lemon juice, grated carrot, and yeast, if using. Cover and blend until totally smooth (this is essential and will take several minutes). Transfer to a covered container and chill until thickened, 2 to 3 hours.

Per 1 tablespoon: 7 calories; 0.2 g protein; 1 g carbohydrate; 0.2 g fat; 0.1 g fiber; 34 mg sodium; calories from protein: 11%; calories from carbohydrates: 57%; calories from fats: 32%

● ● ●

Brown Gravy

MAKES ABOUT 2 CUPS

This traditional-tasting gravy is low in fat and delicious on potatoes, rice, or vegetables.

2 cups water or vegetable broth

1 tablespoon cashews

1 tablespoon onion powder

½ teaspoon garlic granules or powder

2 tablespoons cornstarch

3 tablespoons reduced-sodium soy sauce

Combine all ingredients in blender container. Blend until completely smooth, 2 to 3 minutes.

Transfer to a saucepan and cook over medium heat, stirring constantly, until thickened.

Per ¼-cup serving: 23 calories; 1 g protein; 4 g carbohydrate; 0.5 g fat; 0.1 g fiber; 190 mg sodium; calories from protein: 15%; calories from carbohydrates: 65%; calories from fats: 20%

● ● ●

Quick Bean Dip

MAKES ABOUT 2 CUPS

Serve this dip with baked tortilla chips or use it as a burrito filling. Instant bean flakes (see Glossary) are sold in natural food stores and some supermarkets.

1 cup instant bean flakes
1 cup boiling water

½ to 1 cup salsa (you choose the heat)

Mix bean flakes with boiling water and let stand for 5 minutes. Stir in salsa to taste.

Per ¼-cup serving: 63 calories; 4 g protein; 12 g carbohydrate; 0.2 g fat; 4 g fiber; 117 mg sodium; calories from protein: 25%; calories from carbohydrates: 72%; calories from fats: 3%

● ● ●

Peanut Sauce

MAKES ½ CUP

Peanut sauce is delicious on cooked vegetables and grains. Be aware that it is high in fat and sodium and should be used sparingly.

¼ cup peanut butter
1 tablespoon seasoned rice vinegar
1 tablespoon reduced-sodium soy sauce

1 teaspoon sugar or other sweetener
¾ teaspoon powdered ginger
¼ teaspoon cayenne
¼ cup water

Whisk all ingredients together. Sauce should be thick but pourable. If it is too thick, add water, a teaspoon at a time, until desired consistency is reached.

Per 1 tablespoon: 54 calories; 2 g protein; 3 g carbohydrate; 4 g fat; 0.5 g fiber; 131 mg sodium; calories from protein: 15%; calories from carbohydrates: 22%; calories from fats: 63%

● ● ●

Pineapple Apricot Sauce

MAKES ABOUT 3 CUPS

Use this sauce as a spread on toast or as a topping for cake. It is delicious with Quick and Easy Brown Bread (page 219). It is thickened with agar, a sea vegetable thickener that is sold in natural food stores and Asian markets.

1 cup apple juice concentrate
1½ teaspoons agar powder
1 cup water
1 cup chopped apricots, fresh,
    frozen, or canned

1 8-ounce can crushed pineapple,
    packed in pineapple juice
¼ teaspoon ginger

Combine apple juice and agar with the water in a saucepan. Let stand 5 minutes. Bring to a simmer, stirring occasionally, and cook 3 minutes.

Add apricots, pineapple with its juice, and ginger. Stir to mix. Remove from heat and chill thoroughly, 3 to 4 hours.

Per 1 tablespoon: 13 calories; 0.08 g protein; 3 g carbohydrate;
0 .05 g fat; 0.1 g fiber; 2 mg sodium; calories from protein: 3%;
calories from carbohydrates: 94%; calories from fats: 3%

• • •

Applesauce
MAKES ABOUT 6 CUPS

Homemade applesauce is quite simple to prepare and full of flavor. It can be served hot or cold, or used as a topping for toast, pancakes, or cereal. Directions are given for cooking it on the stove or in a Crock-Pot.

6 large tart apples (gravenstein,
    Pippin, Granny Smith, etc.)
1 cup undiluted apple juice
    concentrate

½ teaspoon cinnamon

For chunky applesauce, peel apples, then core and dice. Place in a large pan. Add apple juice concentrate, then cover and cook over low heat, stirring often, until apples are soft. Mash slightly with a fork if desired, then stir in cinnamon.

For smoother applesauce, cut apples into quarters and remove cores. Chop finely in a food processor. Transfer to a pan and add apple juice concentrate and cinnamon. Cover and cook, stirring often, over low heat until tender, about 15 minutes.

Crock-Pot method: Place diced or chopped apples in Crock-Pot with ½ cup apple juice concentrate and cinnamon. Cover and cook on high for 2½ to 3 hours.

Per ½-cup serving: 101 calories; 0.3 g protein; 26 g carbohydrate; 0.5 g
fat; 2 g fiber; 6 mg sodium; calories from protein: 1%; calories from carbohydrates: 95%; calories from fats: 4%

• • •

Strawberry Sauce

MAKES ABOUT 3 CUPS

Use this sauce on bread or toast or as a topping on pancakes. Agar is a thickener made from a sea vegetable that can be used in place of animal gelatin. It is sold in natural food stores and Asian markets.

1 cup water
1 cup apple juice concentrate
3 cups fresh or frozen strawberries

1½ teaspoons agar powder
1 tablespoon lemon juice

Combine water, apple juice concentrate, 2 cups of the strawberries, and agar in a blender. Process until fairly smooth.

Transfer to a pan. Bring to a simmer, stirring occasionally, and cook 3 minutes. Remove from heat.

Add remaining 1 cup berries, along with lemon juice. Stir to mix. Chill until set, at least 3 hours.

Per 1 tablespoon: 15 calories; 0.09 g protein; 4 g carbohydrate; 0.06 g fat; 0.2 g fiber; 2 mg sodium; calories from protein: 2%; calories from carbohydrates: 94%; calories from fats: 4%

SOUPS AND STEWS

Vegetable Broth

MAKES ABOUT 2 QUARTS

A steamy cup of this broth makes a warm and comforting start to a meal. It may also be used as an ingredient in recipes that call for broth or stock.

1 onion, chopped
1 carrot, chopped
1 celery stalk, chopped
¼ cup chopped fresh parsley
6 cups water
2 teaspoons onion powder
½ teaspoon dried thyme

¼ teaspoon dried turmeric
¼ teaspoon garlic powder
¼ teaspoon dried marjoram
½ teaspoon salt
1 15-ounce can garbanzo beans, including liquid

Combine onion, carrot, celery, parsley, water, onion powder, thyme, turmeric, garlic powder, marjoram, and salt in a large pot. Cover and simmer 20 minutes.

Stir in garbanzo beans with their liquid. Transfer to a blender in small batches and process until completely smooth, about 1 minute per batch. Be sure to hold the lid on tightly and start the blender on the lowest speed.

Per 1-cup serving: 80 calories; 3 g protein; 16 g carbohydrate;
1 g fat; 3 g fiber; 302 mg sodium; calories from protein: 15%;
calories from carbohydrates: 77%; calories from fats: 8%

• • •

Split Pea Soup
MAKES 12 1-CUP SERVINGS

This simple soup contains no added fat and is a perfect warm-up for a cold day. If you are away from home during the day, use the Crock-Pot method and you'll have delicious, hot soup awaiting your return.

2 cups split peas, rinsed
6 cups water or Vegetable Broth
   (page 195)
1 medium onion, chopped
1 large carrot, sliced or diced
2 celery stalks, sliced
1 large potato, peeled and diced
1 large yam, peeled and diced
   (optional)

2 garlic cloves, minced
½ teaspoon dried marjoram
½ teaspoon dried basil
¼ teaspoon ground cumin
¼ teaspoon black pepper
1 teaspoon salt

Combine peas, water, onion, carrot, celery, potato, yam (if using), garlic, marjoram, basil, cumin, and black pepper in a large pot. Simmer, loosely covered, until peas are tender, about 1 hour. Transfer about 4 cups to a blender and purée, starting blender on low speed and holding lid on tightly. Return to pot and stir in salt to taste.

Crock-Pot method: Combine all ingredients in a Crock-Pot and cook on high until peas are tender, about 6 to 8 hours. For quicker cooking, bring water to a boil before adding it to the Crock-Pot.

Per 1-cup serving: 168 calories; 9 g protein; 33 g carbohydrate;
0.5 g fat; 4.5 g fiber; 191 mg sodium; calories from protein: 21%;
calories from carbohydrates: 76%; calories from fats: 3%

• • •

Alphabet Soup
MAKES 8 1-CUP SERVINGS

Little pasta in alphabet shapes makes this soup fun way as well as nourishing.

2 teaspoons olive oil
1 small onion, chopped
2 garlic cloves, minced
4 cups tomato juice
1 small potato, scrubbed and cut
   into chunks
1 carrot, cut into chunks
1 stalk celery, sliced, including top

2 teaspoons Italian herbs
⅛ teaspoon black pepper
½ cup alphabet pasta or small pasta
   shells
1 cup finely chopped spinach,
   kale, or collard greens
1 15-ounce can kidney beans

Heat oil in a large pot and add onion and garlic. Cook over medium-high heat until onion is soft, about 5 minutes.

Add tomato juice, potato, carrot, celery, Italian herbs, and black pepper. Cover and simmer until vegetables are tender, about 20 minutes.

Add pasta, chopped greens, and kidney beans with their liquid. Simmer until greens and pasta are tender, about 15 minutes. Extra tomato juice or water may be added if a thinner soup is desired.

Per 1-cup serving: 128 calories; 5 g protein; 25 g carbohydrate;
1.5 g fat; 6 g fiber; 203 mg sodium; calories from protein: 16%;
calories from carbohydrates: 74%; calories from fats: 10%

● ● ●

Tomato Soup
MAKES ABOUT 6 1-CUP SERVINGS

Tomato Soup provides a delicious warm-up for cold winter days. Serve it with bread or muffins and a salad. For a heartier soup, add a bit of cooked brown rice.

1 onion, chopped
3 stalks celery, sliced, including
   tops
1 28-ounce can crushed tomatoes
1 cup water or Vegetable Broth
   (page 195)
2 tablespoons apple juice
   concentrate

½ teaspoon paprika
½ teaspoon dried basil
¼ teaspoon black pepper
1 tablespoon olive oil
2 tablespoons flour
2 cups fortified soy milk or rice
   milk

Combine onion, celery, crushed tomatoes, water, apple juice concentrate, paprika, basil, and black pepper in a pot. Cover and simmer 15 minutes.

Transfer to a blender in two or three small batches and purée until very smooth, then return to the pot.

In a separate pan, combine oil and flour (it will be very thick). Cook over low heat, stirring constantly for 1 minute. Whisk in milk and cook over medium heat, stirring frequently until steamy and slightly thickened, about 5 minutes. Add to tomato mixture and stir to mix.

Per 1-cup serving: 105 calories; 4 g protein; 15 g carbohydrate;
4 g fat; 3 g fiber; 245 mg sodium; calories from protein: 15%;
calories from carbohydrates: 51%; calories from fats: 34%

• • •

Potato Vegetable Soup
MAKES 8 1-CUP SERVINGS

3 medium potatoes, scrubbed and cut into ½-inch dice
2 stalks celery, sliced
1 large carrot, sliced
2 cups shredded green cabbage

3 cups water
1 cup unsweetened fortified soy milk or rice milk
¾ teaspoon salt
¼ teaspoon black pepper

Combine potatoes, celery, carrot, and cabbage in a large pot with the water. Bring to a simmer, then cover and cook until vegetables are tender, about 15 minutes.

Transfer about 3 cups of the mixture to a blender. Add milk, salt, and pepper. Hold lid on tightly and blend until completely smooth, about 30 seconds, then return to the pot and stir to mix. Heat gently before serving.

Per 1-cup serving: 99 calories; 2.5 g protein; 22 g carbohydrate;
0.3 g fat; 3 g fiber; 221 mg sodium; calories from protein: 10%;
calories from carbohydrates: 87%; calories from fats: 3%

• • •

Lentil Barley Stew
MAKES 6 1-CUP SERVINGS

This hearty one-step stew makes a complete meal when it is served with a crisp green salad.

½ cup lentils, rinsed
¼ cup hulled or pearled barley
4 cups Vegetable Broth (page 195) or water
1 small onion, chopped
1 garlic clove, pressed or minced
1 carrot, diced

1 celery stalk, sliced
½ teaspoon dried oregano
½ teaspoon ground cumin
¼ teaspoon red pepper flakes
¼ teaspoon black pepper
½ to 1 teaspoon salt

Place all ingredients except salt in a large pot and bring to a simmer. Cover and cook, stirring occasionally, until lentils and barley are tender, about 1 hour. Add salt to taste.

Per 1-cup serving: 132 calories; 7 g protein; 26 g carbohydrate;
0.3 g fat; 5 g fiber; 230-460 mg sodium; calories from protein: 21%;
calories from carbohydrates: 76%; calories from fats: 3%

● ● ● ●

Broccoli Potato Soup

MAKES ABOUT 6 1-CUP SERVINGS

Broccoli is a nutritional powerhouse, and this creamy soup makes it appealing to children.

2½ cups Vegetable Broth (page 195), divided
1 onion, chopped
2 garlic cloves, minced
2 potatoes, diced
4 cups broccoli florets
½ teaspoon cumin

½ teaspoon salt
¼ teaspoon black pepper
1 tablespoon tahini (sesame butter)
2 cups fortified unsweetened soy milk

Heat ½ cup of the vegetable broth in a large pot, then add onion and garlic and cook, stirring occasionally until soft, about 5 minutes.

Add diced potatoes and remaining 2 cups broth, then cover and simmer until potatoes are tender, about 15 minutes.

Add broccoli and simmer until tender, about 5 minutes. Stir in cumin, salt, pepper, and tahini.

Transfer small batches to a blender and purée until very smooth, adding some of the soy milk to each batch. Return to pot and warm over low heat until steamy.

Per 1-cup serving: 140 calories; 5 g protein; 27 g carbohydrate;
2 g fat; 5 g fiber; 373 mg sodium; calories from protein: 14%;
calories from carbohydrates: 72%; calories from fats: 14%

● ● ● ●

Pumpkin Soup

MAKES ABOUT 8 1-CUP SERVINGS

This sweet and creamy soup has just a hint of spiciness. It can also be made with pureed winter squash, yams, or sweet potatoes in place of the pumpkin.

1   tablespoon olive oil
1   onion, chopped
2   garlic cloves, minced
½   teaspoon mustard seeds
½   teaspoon turmeric
½   teaspoon ground ginger
½   teaspoon ground cumin
¼   teaspoon cinnamon
¾   teaspoon salt

2   cups water or Vegetable Broth
    (page 195)
1   15-ounce can pumpkin
2   tablespoons maple syrup or
    other sweetener
1   tablespoon lemon juice
2   cups fortified soy milk or rice
    milk

Warm oil in a large pot. Add onion and garlic and cook over medium heat until onion is soft, about 5 minutes.

Add mustard seeds, turmeric, ginger, cumin, cinnamon, and salt and cook 2 minutes over medium heat, stirring constantly.

Whisk in water or broth, pumpkin, maple syrup, and lemon juice. Simmer 15 minutes.

Remove from heat and stir in milk. Transfer about 3 cups to a blender and purée until very smooth. Repeat with remaining soup. Be sure to start on low speed and hold lid on tightly. Return to the pot and heat without boiling, until steamy.

Per 1-cup serving: 78 calories; 3 g protein; 11 g carbohydrate;
3 g fat; 3 g fiber; 211 mg sodium; calories from protein: 14%;
calories from carbohydrates: 55%; calories from fats: 31%

ENTRÉES

Very Primo Pasta

MAKES 10 1-CUP SERVINGS

Pasta with beans, an Italian favorite, is simple and satisfying!

½   cup water or Vegetable Broth
    (page 195)
1   onion, chopped
1   bell pepper, seeded and diced
1   carrot, sliced
1   stalk celery, sliced
2   cups sliced mushrooms (about
    ½ pound)

1   15-ounce can chopped tomatoes
1   15-ounce can kidney beans,
    drained
½   teaspoon paprika
½   teaspoon black pepper
1   tablespoon low-sodium soy
    sauce
8   ounces rigatoni or similar pasta

In a large pot, heat water or broth. Cook onions over high heat until soft, about 5 minutes.

Reduce heat to medium and add pepper, carrot, and celery. Cook 5 minutes.

Add mushrooms, cover and cook 7 minutes, stirring occasionally.

Add tomatoes, kidney beans, paprika, black pepper, and soy sauce. Cover and cook 10 to 15 minutes.

Cook pasta according to package directions. Drain and rinse, then add to sauce.

Per 1-cup serving: 154 calories; 7 g protein; 30 g carbohydrate;
1 g fat; 6 g fiber; 128 mg sodium; calories from protein: 18%;
calories from carbohydrates: 78%; calories from fats: 4%

• • •

Terrific Tacos
MAKES 10 TO 12 TACOS

Textured vegetable protein (TVP) is an inexpensive soy product that makes one of the tastiest tacos around. Look for it in natural food stores and some supermarkets.

1 small onion, chopped	1 tablespoon reduced-sodium soy
2 garlic cloves, minced or pressed	sauce
½ small bell pepper, finely diced	12 corn tortillas
¾ cup textured vegetable protein	1 cup shredded romaine lettuce
1 cup tomato sauce	4 green onions, sliced
2 teaspoons chili powder	1 medium tomato, diced
½ teaspoon cumin	1 avocado, cut into strips
¼ teaspoon oregano	(optional)
1 tablespoon nutritional yeast	½ cup salsa or taco sauce
(optional)	

Heat ½ cup water in a large pot or skillet. Cook onion, garlic, and bell pepper until soft, about 5 minutes.

Add textured vegetable protein, 1 cup water, tomato sauce, chili powder, cumin, oregano, nutritional yeast (if using), and soy sauce. Cook over low heat until mixture is fairly dry, about 15 minutes.

Heat a tortilla in a dry skillet until soft and pliable. Top with about ¼ cup of filling and fold in half. Cook 1 minute on each side. Garnish with lettuce, onions, tomato, avocado, and salsa. Repeat with remaining tortillas.

Per taco: 112 calories; 5 g protein; 17 g carbohydrate; 3 g fat;
3 g fiber; 213 mg sodium; calories from protein: 17%;
calories from carbohydrates: 58%; calories from fats: 25%

• • •

Sloppy Joes

MAKES 4 SERVINGS

This healthy version of a childhood favorite is a hit with old and young alike.

1 large onion, finely chopped	1 teaspoon garlic powder or
1 red bell pepper, seeded and	granules
finely diced	2 tablespoons cider vinegar
1 cup textured vegetable protein	1 tablespoon reduced-sodium soy
1 15-ounce can tomato sauce	sauce
2 tablespoons apple juice concen-	1 teaspoon stone-ground or Dijon
trate	mustard
1 teaspoon chili powder	4 whole wheat burger buns

Heat 1/2 cup water in a large pot. Add onion and bell pepper and cook over high heat until soft, about 5 minutes. Add textured vegetable protein, 1 cup water, tomato sauce, apple juice concentrate, chili powder, garlic powder, vinegar, soy sauce, and mustard. Cook over medium heat, stirring frequently, until thick, about 10 minutes.

Cut buns in half and warm in a toaster oven. Top each half with about 1/2 cup of sauce.

Per 1 bun plus 1 cup sauce: 248 calories; 14 g protein; 46 g carbohydrate;
2 g fat; 8 g fiber; 1062 mg sodium; calories from protein: 21%;
calories from carbohydrates: 69%; calories from fats: 10%

● ● ●

Fast Lane Chow Mein

MAKES 6 1-CUP SERVINGS

This chow mein takes just minutes to prepare and is a delicious way to load up on nutritious vegetables. Ramen soups are sold in natural food stores and many supermarkets. Be sure to choose a vegetarian brand in which the noodles are baked rather than fried. Westbrae and Soken are two such brands.

1 small onion, chopped	1/2 cup thinly sliced green cabbage
2 garlic cloves, minced	1 cup chopped bok choy or
1 celery stalk, thinly sliced	broccoli florets
1 cup sliced mushrooms (about	2 packages vegetarian ramen soup
1/4 pound)	

Heat 1/2 cup water in a large pot. Add onion and garlic and cook until onion is soft, about 5 minutes.

Add celery, mushrooms, cabbage, and bok choy or broccoli.

Break ramen noodles into pieces and add to vegetables along with one of the ramen seasoning packets and 1 cup water. Stir to mix, then cover and cook over medium-high heat until vegetables and noodles are tender, 5 to 7 minutes. Stir occasionally and add a bit more water if mixture begins to stick.

> Per 1-cup serving: 113 calories; 5 g protein; 24 g carbohydrate;
> 0.1 g fat; 2 g fiber; 169 mg sodium; calories from protein: 18%;
> calories from carbohydrates: 81%; calories from fats: 1%

• • •

Spaghetti

MAKES ABOUT 8 1-CUP SERVINGS

Yves Veggie Ground Round takes the place of meat in this simple spaghetti recipe. You could also use Harvest Burger for recipes, Gimme Lean, or crumbled Boca Burgers.

2 teaspoons olive oil	2 teaspoons mixed Italian herbs
1 small onion, chopped	¼ teaspoon black pepper
2 garlic cloves, pressed	2 tablespoons apple juice
1 15-ounce can crushed or stewed	concentrate
tomatoes	6 to 8 ounces spaghetti, preferably
1 package Yves Veggie Ground	whole wheat
Round	

Heat oil in a large pot or skillet. Add onion and garlic and cook until soft, about 5 minutes. Add tomatoes, Veggie Ground Round, Italian herbs, black pepper, and apple juice concentrate. Simmer until flavors are blended, about 15 to 20 minutes.

Cook spaghetti in boiling water according to package directions. Drain and rinse. Add to sauce, and stir to mix.

> Per 1-cup serving: 169 calories; 10 g protein; 28 g carbohydrate;
> 2 g fat; 5 g fiber; 121 mg sodium; calories from protein: 23%;
> calories from carbohydrates: 68%; calories from fats: 9%

• • •

Peanut Butter Spaghetti

MAKES 4 1-CUP SERVINGS

Peanut sauce takes just minutes to prepare and gives spaghetti a whole new personality. Serve this spaghetti with lightly steamed vegetables.

8   ounces uncooked spaghetti
½ cup peanut butter
1   cup hot water
2   tablespoons reduced-sodium soy
    sauce

2   tablespoons seasoned rice
    vinegar
1   tablespoon sugar or other
    sweetener
2   garlic cloves, minced
½ teaspoon powdered ginger

Cook spaghetti according to package directions. Drain, rinse, and set aside.

In a saucepan large enough to hold the pasta, combine peanut butter, water, soy sauce, vinegar, sugar, garlic, and ginger. Whisk until smooth.

Heat gently until slightly thickened. Add cooked pasta and toss to mix. Serve immediately.

Per 1-cup serving: 302 calories; 12 g protein; 30 g carbohydrate;
16 g fat; 4 g fiber; 520 mg sodium; calories from protein: 14%;
calories from carbohydrates: 39%; calories from fats: 47%

● ● ●

Manicotti
MAKES 8 TO 10 SERVINGS

Tofu makes a delicious creamy filling for manicotti. For the best texture and flavor, use firm tofu that is very fresh.

The Sauce:
1   onion, chopped
4   garlic cloves, pressed or minced
3   cups sliced mushrooms (about
    ¾ pound)
½ cup chopped fresh parsley
1   28-ounce can crushed or ground
    tomatoes
3   tablespoons apple juice
    concentrate
1   teaspoon dried basil
1   teaspoon dried oregano
½ teaspoon fennel seeds (optional)
¼ teaspoon black pepper

The Filling:
½ cup chopped fresh parsley
1   garlic clove
1   pound firm tofu
1   teaspoon dried basil
½ teaspoon dried oregano
½ teaspoon dried thyme
½ teaspoon ground nutmeg
½ teaspoon salt
¼ teaspoon black pepper

8 to 10 uncooked manicotti
    shells

To prepare sauce, heat ½ cup water in a large pot. Add onion and garlic and cook until soft, about 5 minutes.

Add mushrooms and parsley. Lower heat slightly, cover and cook until mushrooms are soft, about 5 minutes.

Stir in tomatoes, apple juice concentrate, 1 cup water, basil, oregano, fennel seeds, and black pepper. Cover and simmer 15 minutes, stirring occasionally.

To prepare filling, chop parsley and garlic in a food processor, then add tofu, basil, oregano, thyme, nutmeg, salt, and black pepper. Process until smooth.

Preheat oven to 350°F.

Spread 1 cup of tomato sauce in a 9-by-13-inch (or larger) baking dish. Stuff uncooked manicotti shells with tofu mixture and arrange in baking dish.

Spread with remaining tomato sauce and cover pan tightly with foil. Bake until shells are soft, about 1 hour.

Per manicotti: 155 calories; 8 g protein; 26 g carbohydrate;
3 g fat; 3 g fiber; 246 mg sodium; calories from protein: 20%;
calories from carbohydrates: 64%; calories from fats: 16%

● ● ●

Beanie Weenies
MAKES 6 1-CUP SERVINGS

This old campfire favorite is easy to prepare at home.

2 or 3 Yves Veggie Wieners or other meatless hot dogs	2 cups Baked Beans (page 208) or 1 16-ounce can vegetarian baked beans

Cut hot dogs into ¼-inch-thick slices and place into a saucepan. Add baked beans and cook over medium heat, stirring occasionally, until beans begin to simmer.

Per 1-cup serving: 158 calories; 15 g protein; 22 g carbohydrate;
4.5 g fat; 2 g fiber; 577 mg sodium; calories from protein: 36%;
calories from carbohydrates: 55%; calories from fats: 9%

● ● ●

Hearty Chili Mac
MAKES 10 1-CUP SERVINGS

Children of all ages will enjoy this tasty combination of chili and pasta.

8 ounces macaroni	1 28-ounce can crushed tomatoes
1 onion, chopped	1 15-ounce can kidney beans
3 garlic cloves, minced	1 15-ounce can corn
1 small red or green bell pepper, seeded and diced	2 tablespoons chili powder
	1 teaspoon ground cumin
1 package Yves Veggie Ground Round or 4 Boca Burgers, thawed and chopped	

Cook pasta in boiling water until it is tender. Drain, rinse, and set aside.

Heat ½ cup water in a large pot. Add chopped onion and garlic. Cook until onion is soft, about 5 minutes.

Add bell pepper and Veggie Ground Round or chopped burgers. Mix in crushed tomatoes, kidney beans and corn with their liquids, chili powder, and cumin. Cover and simmer over medium heat, stirring occasionally, for 20 minutes.

Add cooked pasta and check seasonings. Add more chili powder if a spicier dish is desired.

Per 1-cup serving: 156 calories; 10 g protein; 29 g carbohydrate;
1 g fat; 6 g fiber; 432 mg sodium; calories from protein: 24%;
calories from carbohydrates: 71%; calories from fats: 5%

● ● ●

Neat Loaf

MAKES 12 SLICES

Neat Loaf is loaded with healthy vegetables, whole grains, and soy. Serve it with Mashed Potatoes (page 215) and Brown Gravy (page 192) for meal that will make everyone happy. The vegetables should be very finely chopped, a task easily accomplished with a food processor.

1 cup cooked Brown Rice (page 176)	3 tablespoons reduced-sodium soy sauce
2 cups bread crumbs	2 teaspoons stone-ground or Dijon mustard
1 cup walnuts, finely chopped	¼ teaspoon black pepper
1 small onion, finely chopped	vegetable oil cooking spray
2 celery stalks, finely chopped	additional barbecue sauce or ketchup
1 carrot, finely chopped	
1 pound firm tofu	
¼ cup barbecue sauce	

Preheat oven to 350°F.

In a large bowl, combine rice, bread crumbs, walnuts, onion, celery, and carrot.

Puree tofu in a food processor, or mash by hand until very smooth. Add to rice mixture along with barbecue sauce, soy sauce, mustard, and black pepper.

Stir with a large spoon or knead mixture by hand until it is well mixed and holds together, about 1 minute.

Transfer to an oil-sprayed 5-by-9-inch loaf pan or other baking dish and distribute evenly using a spoon, spatula, or your hand.

Top with barbecue sauce or ketchup. Bake 60 minutes. Let stand 10 minutes before serving.

Variation: Leftover Neat Loaf makes a quick and delicious sandwich. Simply arrange a slice of cold Neat Loaf on whole wheat bread with lettuce, tomato, and your favorite condiment, such as vegan mayonnaise, mustard, ketchup, or barbecue sauce.

Per slice: 154 calories; 6 g protein; 15 g carbohydrate;
8 g fat; 2 g fiber; 572 mg sodium; calories from protein: 16%;
calories from carbohydrates: 37%; calories from fats: 48%

Per sandwich: 316 calories; 13 g protein; 42 g carbohydrate;
12 g fat; 5 g fiber; 652 mg sodium; calories from protein: 15%;
calories from carbohydrates: 52%; calories from fats: 33%

●　●　●

Polenta with Spicy Tofu
MAKES 4 SERVINGS

This spicy tofu sauce may also be served over warmed burger buns or cooked brown rice.

1 tablespoon olive oil	2 to 3 teaspoons chili powder
1 large onion, chopped	1 teaspoon garlic granules or
1 red or green bell pepper, seeded and finely diced	powder
	2 tablespoons cider vinegar
1 pound firm tofu, coarsely chopped	1 tablespoon soy sauce
	1 teaspoon stone-ground
1 15-ounce can tomato sauce or crushed tomatoes	mustard
	4 cups cooked Polenta (page 178)
1 tablespoon sugar or other sweetener	

Heat oil in a large pot or skillet. Add onion and bell pepper and cook until soft, about 5 minutes.

Stir in tofu and continue cooking, stirring often, 5 minutes.

Stir in tomato sauce, sugar, chili powder, garlic granules, vinegar, soy sauce, and mustard. Cover and cook over medium heat, stirring frequently, 15 minutes.

To serve, spread cooked polenta onto individual plates and top with sauce.

Per 1-cup sauce with 1-cup polenta: 160 calories; 7.5 g protein; 24 g carbohydrate; 5 g fat; 3 g fiber; 406 mg sodium; calories from protein: 18%; calories from carbohydrates: 56%; calories from fats: 26%

●　●　●

Baked Beans

MAKES ABOUT 8 1-CUP SERVINGS

These beans may be "baked," on the stovetop, in the oven, or in a Crock-Pot. The longer they cook, the more delicious they become. The optional "Bakkon yeast" is not the same as "baking yeast." Rather, it is a brand name for torula yeast, which has a distinctive smoky flavor, and is sold in natural food stores.

2½ cups dried navy beans or other small white beans	2 tablespoons vinegar
1 onion, chopped	½ teaspoon garlic granules or powder
1 15-ounce can tomato sauce	1 teaspoon salt
½ cup molasses	1 teaspoon Bakkon yeast (optional)
2 teaspoons stone-ground or Dijon mustard	

Rinse the beans thoroughly, then soak in 6 cups water for 6 to 8 hours or overnight. Discard the soaking water and place the beans and chopped onion in a pot with enough fresh water to cover the beans with 1 inch of liquid. Bring to a simmer, then cover and cook until the beans are tender, about 2 hours.

Add tomato sauce, molasses, mustard, vinegar, garlic granules, salt, and Bakkon yeast (if using). Cook, loosely covered, over very low heat for 1 to 2 hours. Or, transfer to an ovenproof dish and bake covered at 350°F for 2 to 3 hours.

Crock-Pot method: Place cooked beans into a Crock-Pot with remaining ingredients. Cover and cook on high for 2 to 3 hours.

Per 1-cup serving: 166 calories; 6 g protein; 36 g carbohydrate;
0.6 g fat; 6 g fiber; 520 mg sodium; calories from protein: 14%;
calories from carbohydrates: 83%; calories from fats: 3%

● ● ●

Barbecue-Style Baked Tofu

MAKES 6 ¼-INCH-THICK SLICES

The firm texture and delicious flavor of Baked Tofu makes it a perfect snack, sandwich filling, or stir-fry ingredient. Begin with very firm tofu— it should spring back when lightly pressed. If it fails this test, begin by pressing it as directed below. For the marinade, you can use ½ cup of your own favorite barbecue sauce, or follow the recipe.

1 pound firm fresh tofu
¼ cup ketchup
¼ cup apple juice concentrate
2 tablespoons apple cider vinegar
1 tablespoon reduced-sodium soy
  sauce

1 teaspoon onion powder
½ teaspoon garlic powder
¼ teaspoon black pepper
scant pinch cayenne pepper, or
  more to taste

If necessary, press tofu to increase its firmness using the following steps: Line a baking sheet with a clean dishtowel. Cut tofu into 6 equal slices (each slice should be about ¼ inch thick) and place on the dishtowel in a single layer. Cover with a second clean dishtowel, and top with a cutting board. Place several heavy objects (such as canned food, books, jars of beans) on the cutting board. Let stand 30 minutes.

In the meantime, prepare barbecue sauce. Combine ketchup, apple juice concentrate, vinegar, soy sauce, onion and garlic powder, black pepper, and cayenne pepper in a small bowl.

Remove tofu from the press and pat it dry. Carefully arrange slices in a quart-size zip-top plastic bag, then add the sauce. Seal the bag, then carefully massage it so that all the tofu slices are coated with marinade. Refrigerate 4 hours or more (overnight is ideal), turning the bag occasionally to keep all slices coated.

Preheat oven to 375°F. Remove tofu from bag and place it in a glass baking dish. Drizzle with any remaining marinade and bake, uncovered, until dry and deep golden brown, about 35 minutes.

Per slice: 91 calories; 7 g protein; 10 g carbohydrate;
4 g fat; 1 g fiber; 213 mg sodium; calories from protein: 27%;
calories from carbohydrates: 39%; calories from fats: 34%

● ● ●

Quick Chili Beans

MAKES 9 1-CUP SERVINGS

These chili beans are quick to prepare and delicious with Corn Bread (page 218) or Polenta (page 178). Yves Veggie Ground Round adds hearty flavor and texture as well as protein. Similar products include Harvest Burger for Recipes and Gimme Lean Beef Style. You could also use ½ cup of textured vegetable protein (TVP) which has been softened with ½ cup of boiling water, or 2 to 3 crumbled Boca Burgers. You will find these products in natural food stores and many supermarkets.

2   15-ounce cans pinto beans, including liquid

1   15-ounce can tomato sauce

1   4-ounce can diced green chilies

1   8-ounce package Yves Veggie Ground Round, rehydrated TVP, Harvest Burger for Recipes, or similar product

1   tablespoon onion granules or powder

1   teaspoon garlic granules or powder

1   cup corn, fresh, frozen, or canned

½   teaspoon cumin

Combine all ingredients in a pot. Cover and simmer over medium-low heat for 15 minutes, stirring occasionally.

Per 1-cup serving: 132 calories; 10 g protein; 23 g carbohydrate; 0.3 g fat; 6 g fiber; 472 mg sodium; calories from protein: 30%; calories from carbohydrates: 68%; calories from fats: 2%

● ● ●

Tamale Pie

MAKES 12 SERVINGS

Simple chili beans topped with polenta make a delicious golden-crusted pie.

5   cups water

1   cup polenta

1   teaspoon salt

1   large yellow onion, chopped

3   large garlic cloves, minced

1   red or green bell pepper, seeded and diced

1   12-ounce package Yves Veggie Ground Round (or similar product)

1   tablespoon chili powder

1   teaspoon cumin

1   28-ounce can crushed tomatoes

1   15-ounce can vegetarian chili beans

Measure water into a large pot, then whisk in polenta and salt. Simmer over medium-low heat, stirring often, until very thick, about 25 minutes. Set aside.

Heat ½ cup water in a large skillet or pot and add onion, garlic, and bell pepper. Cook until soft, about 5 minutes, stirring occasionally.

Add Veggie Ground Round, chili powder, and cumin. Cook over medium heat, stirring often, 3 minutes. Add a bit more water if needed to prevent sticking.

Stir in tomatoes and chili beans with their liquid. Cover and simmer 10 minutes.

Preheat oven to 350°F.

Transfer to a 9-by-13-inch baking dish. Spread cooked polenta evenly over top. Bake for 20 minutes.

Per serving ($\frac{1}{12}$ of recipe): 104 calories; 7 g protein; 18 g carbohydrate;
0.4 g fat; 5 g fiber; 347 mg sodium; calories from protein: 28%;
calories from carbohydrates: 69%; calories from fats: 3%

VEGETABLES

Broccoli with Golden Sunshine Sauce

MAKES ABOUT 4 1-CUP SERVINGS

Broccoli has been called the king of vegetables for good reason. It is a powerhouse of nutrients including protein, calcium, and iron, and it is delicious bathed in Golden Sunshine Sauce. The sauce is made with nutritional yeast (see Glossary) which gives it a lovely golden glow.

1 bunch broccoli (3 to 4 stalks)
2 tablespoons nonhydrogenated
   margarine

1 tablespoon nutritional yeast

Break broccoli into bite-size florets. Peel stems and slice into $\frac{1}{4}$-inch-thick rounds. Steam until bright green and just tender, about 5 minutes.

While broccoli is steaming, melt margarine in a saucepan. Stir in nutritional yeast. Add steamed broccoli and toss to mix. Serve immediately.

Per 1-cup serving: 80 calories; 4 g protein; 6 g carbohydrate;
6 g fat; 4 g fiber; 78 mg sodium; calories from protein: 16%;
calories from carbohydrates: 24%; calories from fats: 60%

● ● ●

Braised Collards or Kale

MAKES 3 1-CUP SERVINGS

Collard greens and kale are rich sources of calcium and beta-carotene as well as other minerals and vitamins. One of the tastiest—and easiest—ways to prepare them is with a bit of soy sauce and plenty of garlic. Try to purchase young tender greens, as these have the best flavor and texture.

1 bunch collard greens or kale
   (6 to 8 cups chopped)
1 teaspoon olive oil
2 teaspoons reduced-sodium soy
   sauce

1 teaspoon balsamic vinegar
2 to 3 garlic cloves, minced
$\frac{1}{4}$ cup water

Wash greens, remove stems, then cut leaves into ½-inch-wide strips.

Combine olive oil, soy sauce, vinegar, garlic, and water in a large pot or skillet. Cook over high heat about 30 seconds. Reduce heat to medium-high, add chopped greens, and toss to mix. Cover and cook, stirring often, until greens are tender, about 5 minutes.

Per 1-cup serving: 106 calories; 6 g protein; 18 g carbohydrate; 2 g fat; 6 g fiber; 132 mg sodium; calories from protein: 20%; calories from carbohydrates: 60%; calories from fats: 20%

● ● ●

Bok Choy

MAKES 3 1-CUP SERVINGS

Bok choy is another calcium-rich dark leafy green. The stems are crisp and tender, and can be sliced and cooked with the leaves.

2 bunches bok choy (about 6 cups chopped)	2 to 3 garlic cloves, minced
1 teaspoon olive oil	¼ cup water
2 teaspoons reduced-sodium soy sauce	1 teaspoon balsamic vinegar

Wash bok choy, then slice leaves and stems into ½-inch strips.

Combine olive oil, soy sauce, garlic, and water in a large pot or skillet. Cook over high heat about 30 seconds, then add bok choy and toss to mix.

Reduce heat to medium-high, then cover and cook, stirring often, until tender, about 5 minutes. Sprinkle with balsamic vinegar and toss to mix.

Per 1-cup serving: 60 calories; 4 g protein; 8 g carbohydrate; 2 g fat; 2 g fiber; 306 mg sodium; calories from protein: 23%; calories from carbohydrates: 41%; calories from fats: 36%

● ● ●

Summer Squash with Basil

MAKES ABOUT 4 1-CUP SERVINGS

Most markets sell a variety of summer squashes, including green and yellow zucchini, crookneck, and scallop squashes. You may use a single variety or a mixture in this recipe.

2 teaspoons olive oil	½ cup chopped fresh basil
4 medium summer squash, sliced (about 5 cups)	¼ teaspoon salt
	⅛ teaspoon black pepper

Heat oil in a large skillet and add sliced squash. Cover and cook over medium heat, stirring occasionally, until barely tender, about 3 minutes.

Add chopped basil, then cover and cook another 2 to 3 minutes. Sprinkle with salt and pepper.

Per 1-cup serving: 48 calories; 2 g protein; 6 g carbohydrate; 2 g fat; 2 g fiber; 138 mg sodium; calories from protein: 17%; calories from carbohydrates: 42%; calories from fats: 41%

● ● ●

Sesame Asparagus
MAKES 4 1-CUP SERVINGS

The secret to delicious asparagus is cooking it until it is just tender. It should be bright green and still retain a bit of crispness. Be sure to use "toasted" sesame oil, which is dark and very flavorful.

1   pound fresh asparagus   1   tablespoon Sesame Salt
1   teaspoon toasted sesame oil   (page 191)

Trim ends off asparagus, then steam spears until just tender, 3 to 5 minutes.

Place in a serving dish and sprinkle with sesame oil. Toss to coat, then sprinkle with Sesame Salt.

Per 1-cup serving: 54 calories; 4 g protein; 6 g carbohydrate; 2 g fat; 3 g fiber; 36 mg sodium; calories from protein: 22%; calories from carbohydrates: 42%; calories from fats: 36%

● ● ●

Oven Fries
MAKES 4 1-CUP SERVINGS

These delicious oven-roasted potatoes are very low in fat.

2   russet potatoes (about 1 pound)   1   teaspoon paprika
2   teaspoons olive oil   ¼ teaspoon salt

Preheat oven to 450°F. For easy cleanup, line a 9-by-13-inch (or larger) baking dish with baking parchment or foil.

Scrub potatoes, but do not peel. Cut into fries or wedges. Place in a large bowl and toss with oil, paprika, and salt.

Spread in a single layer in the baking dish and bake until tender when pierced with a fork, about 30 minutes.

Per 1-cup serving: 130 calories; 2 g protein; 26 g carbohydrate; 2 g fat; 2 g fiber; 142 mg sodium; calories from protein: 7%; calories from carbohydrates: 77%; calories from fats: 16%

Cooking Potatoes, Sweet Potatoes, Yams, and Winter Squash

Potatoes, sweet potatoes, and winter squash are traditionally baked, but steaming and microwaving are also an excellent methods for cooking these nutritious vegetables. In addition to being quick and easy, the vegetables stay moist and flavorful.

Steaming

To steam potatoes, yams, or sweet potatoes, simply scrub them (or peel them if you prefer) and arrange them on a steamer rack. Cook in a covered pot over simmering water until tender when pierced with a fork. This will take between 15 and 40 minutes, depending on their size. For quicker cooking, cut them into cubes or slices before steaming.

To steam winter squash, cut it in half and scoop out the seeds with a spoon. Cut it into wedges or other conveniently sized pieces and arrange on a steamer rack. Place in a pot, then cover and cook over medium heat until the squash is tender when pierced with a fork, between 15 and 30 minutes, depending on the size and freshness of the squash.

Microwave cooking

Russet Potatoes

2 medium potatoes

Pierce potato in several places with a fork. Place in microwave on rotating surface or turn midway during cooking. Microwave 7 to 8 minutes on high. Pierce with a fork to test for doneness. Crisp potato skins by placing in a toaster oven for a short time.

Sweet Potatoes or Yams

2 medium yams

Place yams in shallow covered casserole. Do not add water. Microwave 6 minutes on high, then turn yams over and microwave another 4 minutes. Test for doneness with a fork.

> *Butternut or Acorn Squash*
>
> 1 squash
>
> Cut squash in half and remove seeds. Place cut side down in a shallow dish. Do not add water. Microwave on high for 8 minutes. Turn squash right side up and cook another 6 minutes on high.

Mashed Potatoes

MAKES ABOUT 10 ½-CUP SERVINGS

Serve with Brown Gravy (page 192) and enjoy this traditional favorite to your heart's content!

4 russet potatoes, peeled and diced	½ teaspoon salt
2 cups water	1½ tablespoons rice flour
1 cup unsweetened fortified soy milk or rice milk	2 tablespoons potato flour
¼ teaspoon onion powder	½ cup Corn Butter (page 191) or 1 tablespoon nonhydrogenated
¼ teaspoon garlic powder	margarine

Put potatoes and water in a saucepan. Simmer until potatoes are tender when pierced with a fork, about 10 minutes. Drain, reserving liquid. Mash potatoes.

Pour milk, onion powder, garlic powder, salt, rice flour, potato flour, and Corn Butter or margarine into a blender. Blend until completely smooth, about 1 minute. Add to mashed potatoes and stir to mix.

Per ½-cup serving: 85 calories; 2 g protein; 18 g carbohydrate; 1 g fat;
2 g fiber; 140 mg sodium; calories from protein: 11%;
calories from carbohydrates: 81%; calories from fats: 8%

● ● ●

Potato Boats

MAKES 4 SERVINGS

Packed full of nutrient-rich broccoli, these potato boats are easy to make and fun to eat.

2 medium potatoes, any variety	1 tablespoon nutritional yeast
2 broccoli stalks	½ teaspoon stone-ground or Dijon mustard
2 tablespoons nonhydrogenated margarine	⅛ teaspoon black pepper

Scrub potatoes and steam until tender when pierced with a fork, about 20 minutes. Remove from pan and cool.

Cut or break broccoli into bite-size florets. Peel stems and slice into ¼-inch-thick rounds (you should have about 2 cups of florets and stems). Steam until just tender, about 5 minutes.

When cool enough to handle, cut potatoes in half lengthwise. Scoop out flesh and place in a food processor. Set shells aside.

Add steamed broccoli to food processor along with margarine, nutritional yeast, mustard, and black pepper. Process until smooth, about 1 minute.

Divide evenly among potato shells.

Preheat oven or toaster oven to 350°F. Place boats in a baking dish and bake, uncovered, 15 minutes.

Microwave method: Place boats in microwave-safe dish and cook on high until heated through, 8 to 10 minutes.

> Per boat: 180 calories; 5 g protein; 29 g carbohydrate;
> 6 g fat; 4 g fiber; 91 mg sodium; calories from protein: 10%;
> calories from carbohydrates: 61%; calories from fats: 29%

● ● ●

Golden Nuggets

ABOUT 4 1-CUP SERVINGS

These oven-roasted sweet potatoes are pure gold. They're nutritious and easy to make and they taste scrumptious. For easy cleanup, line the baking dish with baking parchment or foil.

2 medium sweet potatoes or yams (about 1 pound)	1 teaspoon garlic granules or powder
2 teaspoons olive oil	¼ teaspoon salt
	¼ teaspoon black pepper

Preheat oven to 450°F.

Scrub sweet potatoes and cut into ½-inch chunks. Place in a large bowl and sprinkle with olive oil, garlic granules, salt, and pepper.

Line two 9-by-13-inch baking dishes with baking parchment or foil and add sweet potatoes. Arrange in a single layer.

Bake until tender when pierced with a fork, 25 to 30 minutes.

> Per 1-cup serving: 136 calories; 2 g protein; 28 g carbohydrate;
> 2 g fat; 4 g fiber; 144 mg sodium; calories from protein: 7%;
> calories from carbohydrates: 79%; calories from fats: 14%

● ● ●

Winter Squash with Peanut Sauce

MAKES 6 SERVINGS

Most markets sell a wide variety of delicious winter squashes, with marvelous names like delicata, butternut, kabocha, and sweet dumpling. Each has its characteristic flavor, and all are excellent sources of the antioxidant nutrient beta-carotene. There are a number of ways to cook winter squash, including baking, microwaving, and steaming. In this recipe, the squash is steamed then topped with a flavorful peanut sauce.

3 small winter squash (delicata, sweet dumpling, or similar)	1 tablespoon seasoned rice vinegar
⅓ cup peanut butter	2 teaspoon sugar or other sweetener
⅓ cup hot water	2 garlic cloves, pressed or minced
1 tablespoon reduced-sodium soy sauce	1 teaspoon minced fresh ginger or ¼ teaspoon powdered ginger

Cut squash in half and scoop out seeds. Steam until tender when pierced with a fork, about 20 minutes.

While squash cooks, combine peanut butter, hot water, soy sauce, vinegar, sugar, garlic, and ginger in a small saucepan. Mix with a fork or whisk, then heat gently until sauce is smooth and slightly thickened. Add more water if sauce becomes too thick.

When squash is tender, drizzle with peanut sauce and serve.

Per squash half: 110 calories; 5 g protein; 15 g carbohydrate; 5 g fat; 4 g fiber; 96 mg sodium; calories from protein: 16%; calories from carbohydrates: 50%; calories from fats: 34%

• • •

Garlicky Green Beans

MAKES ABOUT 4 1-CUP SERVINGS

These green beans have a delicious Asian flair.

1 pound fresh green beans	1 tablespoon reduced-sodium soy sauce
2 teaspoons toasted sesame oil	2 tablespoons water
8 large garlic cloves, minced	¼ teaspoon black pepper
2 tablespoons seasoned rice vinegar	

Rinse beans, remove stems, then steam until just tender, about 10 minutes. Set aside.

Heat oil in a nonstick skillet and cook garlic, stirring constantly,

1 minute. Stir in vinegar, soy sauce, water, and cooked beans. Sprinkle with pepper and cook, stirring constantly, until very hot, about 2 minutes.

Per 1-cup serving: 80 calories; 2 g protein; 14 g carbohydrate; 2 g fat; 4 g fiber; 400 mg sodium; calories from protein: 13%; calories from carbohydrates: 62%; calories from fats: 25%

BREADS AND DESSERTS

Corn Bread

MAKES 9 SERVINGS

This delicious, crumbly cornbread is made with barley flour, which is sold in natural food stores and some supermarkets.

1½ cups fortified soy milk or rice milk
1½ tablespoons white or cider vinegar
1 cup cornmeal
1 cup barley flour
2 tablespoons sugar or other sweetener
½ teaspoon salt
1 teaspoon baking powder
½ teaspoon baking soda
2 tablespoons canola oil
vegetable oil cooking spray

Preheat oven to 425°F.

Combine milk and vinegar and set aside.

Mix cornmeal, barley flour, sugar, salt, baking powder, and baking soda in a large bowl.

Add milk mixture and oil. Stir until just blended.

Spread batter evenly in an oil-sprayed 9-by-9-inch baking dish. Bake until top is golden brown, 25 to 30 minutes. Serve hot.

Per serving (⅑ of recipe): 158 calories; 4 g protein; 26 g carbohydrate; 4 g fat; 2 g fiber; 194 mg sodium; calories from protein: 10%; calories from carbohydrates: 66%; calories from fats: 24%

• • •

Garlic Bread

MAKES 1 LOAF (ABOUT 20 SLICES)

Using Corn Butter makes this Garlic Bread low in fat compared with its traditional counterpart.

1 cup Corn Butter (page 191)
1 tablespoon garlic granules or powder (more or less to taste)

1 teaspoon Italian herbs
1 loaf French bread (whole wheat if possible)

Preheat oven to 350°F.

Mix Corn Butter, garlic granules, and Italian herbs.

Slice bread and spread with garlic mixture. Wrap in foil and bake for 20 minutes.

Per slice: 88 calories; 3 g protein; 17 g carbohydrate;
1 g fat; 1 g fiber; 229 mg sodium; calories from protein: 13%;
calories from carbohydrates: 76%; calories from fats: 11%

● ● ●

Quick and Easy Brown Bread
MAKES 1 LOAF (ABOUT 20 SLICES)

This bread is made with healthful whole wheat and contains no added fat or oil. Serve it plain or with Pineapple Apricot Sauce (page 193).

1½ cups fortified soy milk or rice milk
2 tablespoons vinegar
3 cups whole wheat pastry flour

2 teaspoons baking soda
½ teaspoon salt
½ cup molasses
½ cup raisins

Preheat oven to 325°F.

Mix milk with vinegar and set aside.

In a large bowl, combine flour, baking soda, and salt. Stir to mix.

Add milk mixture and molasses. Stir to mix, then stir in raisins. Do not overmix.

Spread evenly in 5-by-9-inch nonstick or oil-sprayed loaf pan (pan should be about half full). Bake 1 hour.

Per slice: 100 calories; 3 g protein; 22 g carbohydrate;
1 g fat; 2 g fiber; 186 mg sodium; calories from protein: 12%;
calories from carbohydrates: 82%; calories from fats: 6%

● ● ●

Pumpkin Spice Muffins
MAKES 10 TO 12 MUFFINS

These moist and delicious fat-free muffins are great for breakfast or afternoon snack.

2 cups whole wheat flour or whole
   wheat pastry flour
½ cup sugar
1 tablespoon baking powder
½ teaspoon baking soda
½ teaspoon salt
½ teaspoon cinnamon

¼ teaspoon ground nutmeg
1 15-ounce can solid-pack
   pumpkin
½ cup water
½ cup raisins
vegetable oil cooking spray

Preheat oven to 375°F.

Mix flour, sugar, baking powder, baking soda, salt, cinnamon, and nutmeg in a large bowl.

Add pumpkin, water, and raisins. Stir until just mixed.

Spoon batter into oil-sprayed muffin cups, filling to just below tops.

Bake 25 to 30 minutes, until tops of muffins bounce back when pressed lightly. Remove from oven and let stand 5 minutes in pan. Remove muffins from pan and cool on a rack. Store cooled muffins in an airtight container.

Per muffin: 131 calories; 3 g protein; 31 g carbohydrate;
0.5 g fat; 4 g fiber; 236 mg sodium; calories from protein: 10%;
calories from carbohydrates: 87%; calories from fats: 3%

• • •

Brownies

MAKES 28 BROWNIES

These brownies are tender and delicious with no added fat and no cholesterol. For a real treat, top them with raspberry jam or preserves.

1 cup whole wheat pastry
   flour
1 cup sugar
⅓ cup cocoa powder
¼ cup Roma, Caffix, or Pero
   (optional)
½ teaspoon baking soda
½ teaspoon salt

½ 12.3-ounce package Mori-Nu
   Lite Silken Tofu, firm or extra
   firm
½ cup fortified soy milk or rice
   milk
1½ teaspoons cider vinegar
1½ teaspoons vanilla extract
vegetable oil cooking spray

Preheat oven to 350°F.

Stir flour, sugar, cocoa, Roma (if using), baking soda, and salt together in a large mixing bowl.

Puree tofu in a food processor or blender until completely smooth, then blend in milk, vinegar, and vanilla.

Add tofu mixture to dry ingredients and stir just enough to mix.

Spread batter into a nonstick or oil-sprayed 9-by-13-inch baking dish. Bake until top springs back when pressed lightly in the center, about 25 minutes. Remove from oven and allow to cool in pan 10 minutes.

Per brownie: 48 calories; 1 g protein; 11 g carbohydrate;
0.3 g fat; 1 g fiber; 65 mg sodium; calories from protein: 9%;
calories from carbohydrates: 85%; calories from fats: 6%

● ● ●

Apple Crisp
MAKES 9 SERVINGS

Choose a tart variety of apple, such as Pippin or Granny Smith, for an especially tasty dessert. For a special treat, top it with vanilla nondairy "ice cream."

4   green apples, peeled and cored
3   tablespoons lemon juice
1   tablespoon sugar
1   teaspoon cinnamon
1½ cups quick-cooking rolled oats

¾ cup walnuts, finely chopped
⅓ cup maple syrup
1 teaspoon vanilla extract
¼ teaspoon salt

Slice apples thinly and spread in a 9-by-9-inch baking dish. Sprinkle with lemon juice, sugar, and cinnamon.

Preheat oven to 350°F.

Combine rolled oats, walnuts, maple syrup, vanilla, and salt in a bowl. Stir to mix, then spread evenly over apples.

Bake until apples are tender when pierced with a knife, about 35 minutes. Let stand 5 to 10 minutes before serving.

Per serving (⅑ of crisp): 192 calories; 4 g protein; 31 g carbohydrate;
7 g fat; 3 g fiber; 62 mg sodium; calories from protein: 8%; calories from
carbohydrates: 60%; calories from fats: 32%

● ● ●

Banana Cake
MAKES 12 SERVINGS

This moist, flavorful cake really doesn't need frosting.

2   cups unbleached flour or whole
    wheat pastry flour
1½ teaspoons baking soda
½ teaspoon salt
4   ripe bananas
1   cup sugar or other sweetener

⅓ cup canola oil
¼ cup water
1 teaspoon vanilla extract
½ cup chopped dates or raisins
   (optional)
vegetable oil cooking spray

Preheat oven to 350°F.

Mix flour, baking soda, and salt.

In a large bowl, mash bananas, then add sugar and oil and beat well. Stir in water and vanilla and mix thoroughly.

Add flour mixture, along with chopped dates, if using, and stir to mix. Spread in an oil-sprayed 9-by-13-inch pan, and bake for 45 to 50 minutes, until a toothpick inserted into the center comes out clean.

Per serving (1/12 of cake): 228 calories; 3 g protein; 46 g carbohydrate; 5 g fat; 4 g fiber; 300 mg sodium; calories from protein: 6%; calories from carbohydrates: 75%; calories from fats: 19%

● ● ●

Pumpkin Pie
MAKES 8 SERVINGS

Your holidays will be complete with this healthful version of traditional pumpkin pie.

1 9-inch Fat-free Pie crust (recipe follows) or commercial pie crust

1/2 cup sugar or other sweetener
4 tablespoons cornstarch
1 teaspoon cinnamon
1/2 teaspoon powdered ginger

1/8 teaspoon ground cloves
1/2 teaspoon salt
1 15-ounce can solid-pack pumpkin
1 tablespoon molasses
1 1/2 cups fortified soy milk or rice milk

Preheat oven to 400°F.

Mix sugar, cornstarch, cinnamon, ginger, cloves, and salt, then blend in pumpkin, molasses, and milk. Pour into crust and bake 15 minutes.

Reduce heat to 350°F and bake 45 minutes longer. Cool before cutting.

Per serving (1/8 of pie with Fat-free Pie Crust): 159 calories; 3 g protein; 35 g carbohydrate; 1 g fat; 4 g fiber; 246 mg sodium; calories from protein: 8%; calories from carbohydrates: 86%; calories from fats: 6%

Per serving (1/8 of pie using commercial crust): 198 calories; 4 g protein; 32 g carbohydrate; 7 g fat; 5 g fiber; 261 mg sodium; calories from protein: 8%; calories from carbohydrates: 62%; calories from fats: 30%

● ● ●

Fat-free Pie Crust

MAKES ONE 9-INCH CRUST

This crust is slightly sweet and chewy. It is much lower in fat and easier to prepare than traditional crumb crusts.

1 cup Grape-Nuts cereal	¼ cup apple juice concentrate (undiluted)

Preheat oven to 350°F. Mix cereal and apple juice concentrate and pat into a 9-inch pie pan. Bake in preheated oven for 8 minutes. Cool before filling.

Per serving (⅛ of crust): 63 calories; 2 g protein; 15 g carbohydrate; 0.08 g fat; 1 g fiber; 97 mg sodium; calories from protein: 10%; calories from carbohydrates: 89%; calories from fats: 1%

● ● ●

Oatmeal Cookies

MAKES 30 2-INCH COOKIES

With the nutrition of a bowl of hot oatmeal and an aroma to soothe the soul, these cookies are a treat to serve with lunch or dinner, or as a healthy afterschool snack.

1 cup unbleached flour or whole wheat pastry flour	¼ cup molasses
½ teaspoon cinnamon	1 teaspoon vanilla extract
½ teaspoon baking soda	1½ cups rolled oats
½ teaspoon baking powder	¼ cup fortified soy milk or rice milk
¼ teaspoon salt	½ cup raisins
½ cup sugar or other sweetener	½ cup chopped walnuts (optional)
⅓ cup vegetable oil	vegetable oil cooking spray

Preheat oven to 350°F.

Mix flour, cinnamon, baking soda, baking powder, and salt in a large bowl.

In a separate bowl, mix sugar, oil, molasses, and vanilla until smooth. Add flour mixture, rolled oats, milk, raisins, and walnuts (if using). Mix well.

Drop by rounded tablespoonfuls onto an oil-sprayed baking sheet, leaving 2 inches between cookies.

Bake until lightly browned, 12 to 15 minutes. Transfer to a rack to cool, then store in an airtight container.

Per cookie (with walnuts): 91 calories; 2 g protein; 13 g carbohydrate;
4 g fat; 1 g fiber; 41 mg sodium; calories from protein: 7%;
calories from carbohydrates: 56%; calories from fats: 37%

Per cookie (without walnuts): 78 calories; 1 g protein; 13 g carbohydrate;
3 g fat; 1 g fiber; 40 mg sodium; calories from protein: 6%;
calories from carbohydrates: 63%; calories from fats: 31%

● ● ●

Chocolate Pudding

MAKES 4 ½-CUP SERVINGS

This delicious, old-fashioned chocolate pudding is sure to be a favorite.

2 cups fortified soy milk or rice
milk
3 tablespoons cocoa

5 tablespoons cornstarch
½ cup sugar
1 teaspoon vanilla extract

Combine milk, cocoa, cornstarch, sugar, and vanilla in a saucepan. Whisk
smooth.

Cook over medium heat, stirring constantly, until pudding is very
thick. Pour into individual serving dishes and chill.

Per ½-cup serving: 172 calories; 2 g protein; 40 g carbohydrate;
1 g fat; 2 g fiber; 2 mg sodium; calories from protein: 5%;
calories from carbohydrates: 88%; calories from fats: 7%

● ● ●

Fruit Gel

MAKES 8 ½-CUP SERVINGS

*This is an all natural alternative to Jell-O! Agar powder and kudzu
("kood-zoo") are natural plant-based thickeners available in natural
food stores.*

1½ cups strawberries, fresh or
frozen
¾ cups apple juice concentrate
½ cup water

½ teaspoon agar powder
1 tablespoon kudzu powder
2 cups blueberries, fresh or
frozen

Chop strawberries by hand or in a food processor.

Place in a pan with apple juice concentrate, water, agar, and kudzu
powder. Stir to mix.

Bring to a simmer and cook 3 minutes, stirring often. Remove from
heat and chill completely.

Fold in blueberries and transfer to serving dishes.

Variations: Two cups of fresh or frozen blackberries or raspberries, or chopped peaches or mango may be substituted for the blueberries.

Per ½-cup serving: 77 calories; 0.5 g protein; 19 g carbohydrate;
0.2 g fat; 2 g fiber; 9 mg sodium; calories from protein: 2%;
calories from carbohydrates: 95%; calories from fats: 3%

• • •

Orange Power Pops
MAKES 8 FROZEN DESSERTS

These creamy frozen treats are a great way to add protein, calcium, potassium, and other nutrients to the diets of finicky eaters.

1   12.3-ounce package Mori-Nu Lite Silken Tofu, firm
1   cup calcium-fortified orange juice concentrate
1   cup fortified vanilla soy milk
¼   cup maple syrup
2   ripe bananas

Combine all ingredients in a blender and process until completely smooth. Pour into ice-pop molds or small paper cups, insert sticks upright, and freeze.

Per piece: 131 calories; 4 g protein; 28 g carbohydrate; 1 g fat;
1 g fiber; 28 mg sodium; calories from protein: 12%;
calories from carbohydrates: 82%; calories from fats: 6%

• • •

Nutty Fruitballs
MAKES ABOUT 30 PIECES

You can vary the flavor of these yummy treats by substituting different fruits.

⅓ cup pitted dates
⅔ cup raisins
⅔ cup golden raisins
⅔ cup dried apricots
⅔ cup dried figs
⅔ cup cashews
½ cup peanut butter
½ cup carob powder

Grind dried fruit and nuts into small pieces in a food grinder or heavy-duty food processor.

Add peanut butter and carob powder, and mix thoroughly.

With wet hands, roll into balls the size of walnuts.

Per fruitball: 86 calories; 2 g protein; 14 g carbohydrate;
3.5 g fat; 2 g fiber; 3 mg sodium; calories from protein: 8%;
calories from carbohydrates: 58%; calories from fats: 34%

BEVERAGES

Banana Oat Shake

MAKES ABOUT 3 1-CUP SERVINGS

Kids love this smooth, creamy shake!

2 medium bananas	2 tablespoons maple syrup
2 cups fortified vanilla soy milk	2 teaspoons vanilla extract
½ cup quick rolled oats	5 or 6 ice cubes

Combine all ingredients in a blender. Process until completely smooth, 2 to 3 minutes. Serve immediately.

> Per 1-cup serving: 193 calories; 5 g protein; 41 g carbohydrate;
> 2 g fat; 4 g fiber; 2.5 mg sodium; calories from protein: 9%;
> calories from carbohydrates: 81%; calories from fats: 10%

● ● ●

Strawberry Smoothie

MAKES ABOUT 2 1-CUP SERVINGS

Try this cold, thick smoothie with whole grain cereal or a muffin for a delicious breakfast. You can buy frozen strawberries or freeze your own in an airtight container. To freeze bananas, peel them and break into inch-long pieces. Pack loosely in an airtight container and freeze. Bananas will keep in the freezer for about two months, strawberries for six months.

1 cup frozen strawberries	½ to 1 cup unsweetened apple juice
1 cup frozen banana chunks	

Place all ingredients in a blender and process on high speed until smooth, 2 to 3 minutes, stopping blender occasionally to move unblended fruit to the center with a spatula. Serve immediately.

> Per 1-cup serving: 121 calories; 3 g protein; 31 g carbohydrate;
> 0.4 g fat; 2 g fiber; 8 mg sodium; calories from protein: 3%;
> calories from carbohydrates: 94%; calories from fats: 3%

Glossary

Foods That May Be New to You

The majority of ingredients in the recipes are common and widely available in grocery stores. A few that may be unfamiliar are described below.

agar a sea vegetable used as a thickener and gelling agent instead of gelatin, an animal by-product. Available in natural food stores and Asian markets. Also may be called "agar agar." Agar comes in several forms, including powder and flakes. The powder is the easiest to measure and the most concentrated form of agar. If a recipe calls for agar flakes and you are using powder, you will have to adjust the amount you use as follows: for each teaspoon of powder called for in the recipe, use approximately 1½ tablespoonfuls of flakes to substitute.

apple juice concentrate frozen concentrate for making apple juice. May be used full strength as a sweetener.

arrowroot a natural thickener that may be substituted for cornstarch.

baked tofu tofu that has been marinated and baked until it is very firm and flavorful. Baked tofu is usually available in a variety of flavors. Sold in natural food stores and many supermarkets (check the deli and produce sections).

Bakkon yeast a type of nutritional yeast with a smoky flavor. Also called "torula yeast." Sold in natural food stores.

balsamic vinegar mellow-flavored wine vinegar that makes delicious salad dressings and marinades. Available in most food stores.

barley flour can be used in baked goods in place of part or all of the wheat flour for a light, somewhat crumbly product. Available in natural food stores and many supermarkets.

Bob's Red Mill products   whole grain flours, multigrain cereal, and baking mixes. Contact the manufacturer to locate a source near you.

Bob's Red Mill Natural Foods, Inc.

5209 S.E. International Way

Milwaukee, OR 97222

800-553-2258

www.bobsredmill.com

Boca Burger   a low-fat vegetarian burger with a meaty taste and texture. Available in natural food stores, usually in the freezer case.

brown rice   an excellent source of protective soluble fiber as well as protein, vitamins, and minerals that are lost in milling white rice. Available in long-grain and short-grain varieties. Long-grain, which is light and fluffy, includes basmati, jasmine, and other superbly flavorful varieties. Short-grain is more substantial and perfect for hearty dishes. Nutritionally there is very little difference between the two. Brown rice is sold in natural food stores and in many supermarkets.

bulgur   hard red winter wheat that has been cracked and toasted. Cooks quickly and has a delicious, nutty flavor. May be sold in supermarkets as "Ala."

carob powder   the roasted powder of the carob bean that can be used in place of chocolate in many recipes. Sold in natural food stores and some supermarkets.

couscous   although it looks like a grain, couscous is actually a very small pasta. Some natural food stores and supermarkets sell a whole wheat version. Look for it in the grain section.

date pieces   pitted, chopped dates that are coated with cornstarch to keep them from sticking together. They are sold in natural food stores and some supermarkets.

diced green chilies   refers to diced Anaheim chilies, which are mildly hot. These are available canned (Ortega is one brand) or fresh. When using fresh chilies, remove the skin by charring it under a broiler and rubbing it off once it has cooled.

Emes Jel   a natural gelling agent made from vegetable ingredients. May be combined with fruit juice to make a natural gelatin.

Fat-Free Nayonaise   a fat-free, cholesterol-free mayonnaise substitute that contains no dairy products or eggs. Sold in natural food stores and some supermarkets.

Fines Herbs   a herb blend that usually features equal parts of tarragon, parsley, and chives, and also may contain chervil. Look for it in the spice section.

garlic granules   another term for garlic powder.

Harvest Burger for Recipes   ready-to-use, ground beef substitute made from soy. Ideal for tacos, pasta sauces, and chili. Made by Green Giant (Pillsbury) and available in supermarket frozen food sections.

instant bean flakes   precooked black or pinto beans that can be quickly reconstituted with boiling water and used as a side dish, dip, sauce, or burrito filling. Fantastic Foods (707-778-7801) and Taste Adventure (Will-Pak Foods, 800-874-0883, www.tasteadventure.com) are two brands available in natural food stores and some supermarkets.

Italian Herbs   a commercially prepared mixture of Italian herbs: basil, oregano, thyme, marjoram, etc. Also may be called "Italian Seasoning." Look for it in the spice section of your market.

jicama ("hick-ama")   a crisp, slightly sweet root vegetable. Usually used raw in salads and with dips, but also may be added to stir-fries. Usually sold in the unrefrigerated area of the produce section.

kudzu ("kood-zoo")   a thickener made from the roots of the kudzu vine, which grows rampantly in the southeastern United States. It is used much like arrowroot or cornstarch and makes a creamy sauce or gel.

miso ("mee-so")   a salty fermented soybean paste used to flavor soup, sauces, and gravies. Available in light, medium, and dark varieties. The lighter-colored versions having the mildest flavor, while the dark are more robust. Sold in natural food stores and Asian markets.

nonhydrogenated margarine   margarine that does not contain hydrogenated oils. Hydrogenated oils raise blood cholesterol and can increase heart disease risk. Three brands of nonhydrogenated margarine are Earth Balance, Canoleo Soft Margarine, and Spectrum Spread.

nori ("nor-ee")   flat sheets of seaweed used for making sushi and nori rolls.

nutritional yeast   a good-tasting yeast that is richly endowed with nutrients, especially B vitamins. Certain nutritional yeasts, such as Red Star Vegetarian Support Formula Nutritional Yeast, are good sources of vitamin B_{12}. Check the label to be sure. Nutritional yeast may be added to foods for its flavor, sometimes described as "cheeselike," as well as for its nutritional value. Look for nutritional yeast in natural food stores.

Pacific Cream Flavored Sauce Base   a nondairy cream soup base made by Pacific Foods of Oregon and sold in natural food stores and many supermarkets.

potato flour   used as a thickener in sauces, puddings, and gravies. One common brand sold in natural food stores and many supermarkets is Bob's Red Mill.

prewashed salad mix, prewashed spinach   mixtures of lettuce, spinach, and other salad ingredients. Because they have been cleaned and dried, they store well and are easy to use. Several different mixes are available in the produce department of most food stores. "Spring mix" is particularly flavorful.

prune puree   may also be called "prune butter." Can be used in place of fat in baked goods. Commercial brands are WonderSlim and Lekvar. Prune baby food or pureed stewed prunes also may be used.

quinoa ("keen-wah")   a highly nutritious grain that cooks quickly and may be served as a side dish, pilaf, or salad. Sold in natural food stores.

red pepper flakes   dried, crushed chili peppers, available in the spice section or with the Mexican foods.

reduced-fat tofu   contains about a third of the fat of regular tofu. Three brands are Mori-Nu Lite, White Wave, and Tree of Life. Sold in natural food stores and supermarkets.

reduced-sodium soy sauce   also may be called "lite" soy sauce. Compare labels to find the brand with the lowest sodium content.

Rice Dream   see "rice milk."

rice flour   a thickener for sauces, puddings, and gravies. Choose white rice flour for the smoothest results. Bob's Red Mill is one common brand sold in natural food stores and many supermarkets.

rice milk   a beverage made from partially fermented rice that can be used in place of dairy milk on cereals and in most recipes. Available in natural food stores and some supermarkets.

roasted red peppers   red bell peppers that have been roasted over an open flame for a sweet, smoky flavor. Roast your own or purchase them already roasted, packed in water, in most grocery stores. Usually located near the pickles.

seasoned rice vinegar   a mild vinegar made from rice and seasoned with sugar and salt. Great for salad dressings and on cooked vegetables. Available in most grocery stores. Located with the vinegar or in the Asian foods section.

seitan ("say-tan")   also called "wheat meat," seitan is a high-protein, fat-free food with a meaty texture and flavor. Available in the deli case or freezer of natural food stores.

silken tofu   a smooth, delicate tofu that is excellent for sauces, cream soups, and dips. Often available in reduced-fat or "lite" versions. One popular brand, Mori-Nu, is widely available in convenient shelf-stable packaging—special packaging that may be stored without refrigeration for up to a year.

soba noodles   spaghetti-like pasta made with buckwheat flour. Has a delicious, distinctive flavor. Sold in natural food stores and in the Asian food section of some supermarkets.

sodium-free baking powder   made with potassium bicarbonate instead of sodium bicarbonate. Sold in natural food stores and some supermarkets. Featherweight is one brand.

soy milk   nondairy milk made from soybeans that can be used in recipes or as a beverage. May be sold fresh, powdered, or in convenient shelf-stable packaging. Choose calcium-fortified varieties. Available in natural food stores and supermarkets.

soy milk powder   can be used in smoothies, baked goods, or mixed with water for a beverage. Choose calcium-fortified varieties. Available in natural food stores and some supermarkets.

Spike   a seasoning mixture of vegetables and herbs. Comes in a salt-free version, as well as the original version, which contains salt. Sold in natural food stores and many supermarkets.

spreadable fruit   natural fruit preserves made of 100 percent fruit with no added sugar.

stone-ground mustard   mustard containing whole mustard seeds. Often contains horseradish.

tahini ("ta-hee-nee")   sesame seed butter. Comes in raw and toasted forms (either will work in the recipes in this book). Sold in natural food stores, ethnic grocery stores, and some supermarkets. Look for it near the peanut butter or with the natural or ethnic foods.

teff   the world's smallest whole grain. Cooks quickly and has a rich, nutty flavor. Delicious as a breakfast cereal. Sold in natural food stores.

textured vegetable protein (TVP)   meatlike ingredient made from defatted soy flour. Rehydrate with boiling water to add protein and meaty texture to sauces, chili, and stews. TVP is sold in natural food stores and in the bulk section of some supermarkets.

tofu   a mild-flavored soy food that is adaptable to many different recipes. Texture varies greatly, from very smooth "silken" tofu to very dense "extra-firm" tofu. Flavor is best when it is fresh, so check freshness date on package.

torula yeast   see "Bakkon yeast."

turbinado sugar   also called "raw sugar" because it is less processed than white sugar.

unbleached flour   white flour that has not been chemically whitened. Available in most grocery stores.

vegetable broth   ready-to-use brands include Pacific Foods, Imagine Foods, and Swanson's. Other brands available in dry form as powder or cubes. Sold in natural food stores and many grocery stores.

wasabe ("wa-sah-bee")   horseradish paste traditionally served with sushi. Sometimes sold fresh, but more commonly sold as a powder to be reconstituted. Look for it where Asian foods are sold.

whole wheat pastry flour   milled from soft spring wheat. Has the nutritional benefits of whole wheat and produces lighter-textured baked goods than regular whole wheat flour. Available in natural food stores.

Yves Veggie Cuisine   meatlike vegetarian products that are fat-free, including burgers, hot dogs, cold cuts, sausages, and Veggie Ground Round. Sold in natural food stores and many supermarkets.

Resources

Cookbooks

Bronfman, David and Rachelle. *Calciyum!* Toronto, Ont., Canada: Bromedia, 1998.

Golbitz, Peter. *Tofu & Soyfoods Cookery.* Summertown, Tenn.: Book Publishing Company, 1998.

Grogan, Bryanna Clark. *20 Minutes to Dinner.* Summertown, Tenn.: Book Publishing Company, 1997.

Melina, Vesanto, and Forest, Joseph. *Cooking Vegetarian.* New York: John Wiley & Sons and Macmillan Canada, 1998.

Raymond, Jennifer. *The Peaceful Palate.* Summertown, Tenn.: Book Publishing Company, 1996.

Solomon, Jay. *150 Vegan Favorites.* Rocklin, Calif.: Prima, 1998.

Stepaniak, Joanne. *Vegan Vittles.* Summertown, Tenn.: Book Publishing Company, 1996.

Warren, Diane; Jones, Susan Smith; and Lindman, Amy Sorvaag. *Vegetable Soup/The Fruit Bowl.* Grants Pass, Ore: Oasis Press, 1997.

Nutrition

Attwood, Charles. *Dr. Attwood's Low-Fat Prescription for Kids.* New York: Penguin Group, 1995.

Davis, Brenda, and Melina, Vesanto. *Becoming Vegan.* Summertown, Tenn.: Book Publishing Company, 2000.

Demas, Antonia. *Food Is Elementary: A Hands-on Curriculum for Young Students.* Ithaca, New York: Food Studies Institute, 1999.

Messina, Virginia, and Messina, Mark. *The Vegetarian Way: Total Health for You and Your Family.* New York: Crown, 1996.

Spock, Benjamin, and Parker, Steven. *Dr. Spock's Baby and Child Care,* 7th ed. New York: Pocket Books, 1998.

Internet

Airplane travel
   http://www.ivu.org/faq/travel.html

Breastfeeding Resources
   http://www.lalecheleague.org

Dining Directories
   http://www.vegdining.com and http://www.vegeats.com/restaurants

Exercise During Pregnancy
   http://www.fitfor2.com

Family Nutrition
   http://www.vegsource.com

Healthy Eating Vegan-Style
   http://www.pcrm.org

Mangels, Reed. *Feeding Vegan Kids*
   http://www.vrg.org/nutshell/kids.htm

Mangels, Reed. *Traveling with Vegan Children*
   http://www.vrg.org/journal/vj97may/976trav.htm

Traveling

The Vegetarian Journal's Guide to Natural Foods Restaurants in the U.S. and Canada. Wayne, N. J.: Avery Publishing Group, 1998; updated every few years.

References

Chapter 1: Healthy Eating Basics

Barnard, R. J.; Lattimore, L.; Holly, R. G.; Cherny, S.; and Pritkin, N. "Response of Non-Insulin-Dependent Diabetic Patients to an Intensive Program of Diet and Exercise." *Diabetes Care* 5 (1982): 370–374.

Barnard, R. J.; Massey, M. R.; Cherny, S.; et al. "Long-Term Use of High-Carbohydrate, High-Fiber and Exercise in the Treatment of NIDDM Patients." *Diabetes Care* 6 (1983): 268–273.

Block, G. "Epidemiologic Evidence Regarding Vitamin C and Cancer." *American Journal of Clinical Nutrition* 54 (1991): 1310S–1314S.

Burr, M. L.; Batese, J.; Fehily, A. M.; and Leger, A. S. "Plasma Cholesterol and Blood Pressure in Vegetarians." *Journal of Human Nutrition* 35 (1981): 437–441.

Burslem, J.; Schonfeld, G.; Howald, M.; Weidman, S. W.; and Miller, J. P. "Plasma Apoprotein and Lipoprotein Lipid Levels in Vegetarians." *Metabolism* 27 (1978): 711–719.

Chang-Claude, J.; Frentzel-Beyme, R.; and Eilber, U. "Mortality Pattern of German Vegetarians after 11 Years of Follow-up." *Epidemiology* 3 (1992): 395–401.

Cooper, R. S.; Goldberg, R. B.; Trevisan, M.; et al. "The Selective Lowering Effect of Vegetarianism on Low Density Lipoproteins in a Crossover Experiment." *Atherosclerosis* 44 (1982): 293–305.

Fisher, M.; Levine, P. H.; Weiner, B.; et al. "The Effect of Vegetarian Diets on Plasma Lipid and Platelet Levels." *Archives of Internal Medicine* 146 (1986): 1193–1197.

Freeland-Graves, J. H.; Bodzy, P. W.; and Eppright, M. A. "Zinc Status of Vegetarians." *Journal of the American Dietetic Association* 77 (1980): 655–661.

Frentzel-Beyme, R.; Claude, J.; and Eilber, U. "Mortality among German Vegetarians: First Results after Five Years of Follow-up." *Nutrition and Cancer* 11 (1988): 117–126.

Guo, W.-D.; Chow, W.-H.; Zheng, W.; Li J.-Y.; and Blot, W. J. "Diet, Serum Markers and Breast Cancer Mortality in China." *Japanese Journal of Cancer Research* 85 (1994): 572–577.

Hardinge, M. G., and Stare, F. J. "Nutrition Studies of Vegetarians." *American Journal of Clinical Nutrition* 2 (1954): 73–82.

Hunninghake, D. B.; Stein, E. A.; Dujovne, C. A.; et al. "The Efficacy of Intensive Dietary Therapy Alone or Combined with Lovastatin in Outpatients with Hypercholesterolemia." *New England Journal of Medicine* 328 (1993): 1213–1219.

Kestin, M.; Rouse, I. L.; Correll, R. A.; and Nestel, P. J. "Cardiovascular Disease Risk Factors in Free-Living Men: Comparison of Two Prudent Diets, One Based on Lacto-Ovo-Vegetarianism and the Other Allowing Lean Meat." *American Journal of Clinical Nutrition* 50 (1989): 280–287.

Lindahl, O.; Lindwall, L.; Spangberg, A.; Stenram, A.; and Ockerman, P. A. "A Vegan Regimen with Reduced Medication in the Treatment of Hypertension." *British Journal of Nutrition* 52 (1984): 11–20.

Margetts, B. M.; Beilin, L. J.; Armstrong, B. K.; and Vandongen, R. "A Randomized Controlled Trial of a Vegetarian Diet in the Treatment of Mild Hypertension." *Clinical and Experimental Pharmacology and Physiology* 12 (1985): 263–266.

Margetts, B. M.; Beilin, L. J.; Vandongen, R.; and Armstrong, B. K. "Vegetarian Diet in Mild Hypertension: A Randomised Controlled Trial." *British Medical Journal* 293 (1986): 1468–1471.

Melby, C. L.; Goldflies, D. G.; Hyner, G. C.; and Lyle, R. M. "Relation between Vegetarian/Nonvegetarian Diets and Blood Pressure in Black and White Adults." *American Journal of Public Health* 79 (1989): 1283–1288.

Melby, C. L.; Hyner, G. C.; and Zoog, B. "Blood Pressure in Vegetarians and Nonvegetarians: A Cross-sectional Analysis." *Nutrition Research* 5 (1985): 1077–1082.

Ophir, O.; Peer, G.; Gilad, J.; Blum, M.; and Aviram, A. "Low Blood Pressure in Vegetarians: The Possible Role of Potassium." *American Journal of Clinical Nutrition* 37 (1983): 755–762.

Ornish, D.; Brown, S. E.; Scherwitz, L. W.; et al. "Can Lifestyle Changes Reverse Coronary Heart Disease?" *Lancet* 336 (1990): 129–133.

Pixley, F.; Wilson, D.; McPherson, K.; and Mann, J. "Effect of Vegetarianism on Development of Gallstones in Women." *British Medical Journal* 29 (1985): 11–12.

Rouse, I. L.; Armstrong, B. K.; Beilin, L. J.; and Vandongen, R. "Blood-Pressure-Lowering Effect of a Vegetarian Diet: Controlled Trial in Normotensive Subjects." *Lancet* 1 (1983): 5–10.

Rouse, I. L.; Armstrong, B. K.; Beilin, L. J.; and Vandongen, R. "Vegetarian Diet, Blood Pressure and Cardiovascular Risk." *Australian and New Zealand Journal of Medicine* 14 (1984): 439–443.

Rouse, I. L.; Belin, L. J.; Mahoney, D. P.; et al. "Nutrient Intake, Blood Pressure, Serum and Urinary Prostaglandins and Serum Thromboxane B_2 in a Controlled Trial with a Lacto-Ovo-Vegetarian Diet." *Journal of Hypertension* 4 (1986): 241–250.

Sacks, F. M.; Ornish, D.; Rosner, B.; McLanahan, S.; Castelli, W. P.; and Kass, E. H. "Plasma Lipoprotein Levels in Vegetarians: The Effect of Ingestion of Fats from Dairy Products." *Journal of the American Medical Association* 254 (1985): 1337–1341.

Snowdon, D. A., and Phillips, R. L. "Does a Vegetarian Diet Reduce the Occurrence of Diabetes?" *American Journal of Public Health* 75 (1985): 507–512.

Thorogood, M.; Carter, R.; Benfield, L.; et al. "Plasma Lipids and Lipoprotein Cholesterol Concentrations in People with Different Diets in Britain." *British Medical Journal* 295 (1987): 351–353.

West, R. O., and Hayes, O. B. "Diet and Serum Cholesterol Levels: A Comparison between Vegetarians and Nonvegetarians in a Seventh-Day Adventist Group." *American Journal of Clinical Nutrition* 21 (1968): 853–862.

Chapter 2: Nutrients and Where to Find Them

Abelow, B. J.; Holford, T. R.; and Insogna, K. L. "Cross-Cultural Association between Dietary Animal Protein and Hip Fracture: A Hypothesis." *Calcified Tissue International* 50 (1992): 14–18.

American Dietetic Association. "Position of the American Dietetic Association: Vegetarian Diets." *Journal of the American Dietetic Association* 97, no. 11 (1997): 1317–1321.

Consumer Reports. "Is Our Fish Fit to Eat?" *Consumer Reports* (February 1992): 103–114.

de Ridder, C. M.; Thijssen, J. H. H.; Vant Veer, P.; et al. "Dietary Habits, Sexual Maturation, and Plasma Hormones in Pubertal Girls: A Longitudinal Study." *American Journal of Clinical Nutrition* 54 (1991): 805–813.

Dwyer, J. T.; Miller, L. G.; Arduino, N. L.; et al. "Mental Age and I.Q. of Predominately Vegetarian Children." *Journal of the American Dietetic Association* 76 (1980): 142–147.

Groff, J. L.; Gropper, S. S.; and Hunt, S. M. *Advanced Nutrition and Human Metabolism.* New York: West, 1995.

Hamilton, E. M. N.; Whitney, E. N.; and Sizer, F. S. *Nutrition Concepts and Controversies,* 6th ed. New York: West, 1994.

Hu, J. F.; Zhao, X. H.; Parpia, B.; and Campbell, T. C. "Dietary Intakes and Urinary Excretion of Calcium and Acids: A Cross-sectional Study of Women in China." *American Journal of Clinical Nutrition* 58 (1993): 389–406.

Krebs-Smith, S. M.; Cook, D. A.; Subar, A. F.; Cleveland, L.; Friday, J.; and Kahle, L. L. "Fruit and Vegetable Intakes of Children and Adolescents in the United States." *Archives of Pediatric and Adolescent Medicine* 150 (1996): 81–86.

Sinha, R.; Rothman, N.; Brown, E. D.; Salmon, C. P.; Knize, M. G.; Swanson, C. A.; Rossi, S. C.; Mark, S. D.; Levander, O. A.; and Felton, J. S. "High Concentrations of the Carcinogen 2-Amino-1-Methyl-6-Phenylimidazo-[4,5-b]Pyridine (PhIP) Occur in Chicken but Are Dependent on the Cooking Method." *Cancer Research* 55, no. 20 (1995): 4516–4519.

Zemel, M. B. "Calcium Utilization: Effect of Varying Level and Source of Dietary Protein." *American Journal of Clinical Nutrition* 48 (1988): 880–883.

Chapter 3: Starting Life Well: Nutrition in Pregnancy

Abrams, B.; Altman, S. L.; and Pickett, K. E. "Pregnancy Weight Gain: Still Controversial." *American Journal of Clinical Nutrition* 71 (2000): 1233S–12341S.

Beaton, G. H. "Iron Needs during Pregnancy: Do We Need to Rethink Our Targets?" *American Journal of Clinical Nutrition* 72 (2000): 265S–2671S.

Buck, G. M.; Vena, J. E.; Schisterman, E. F.; Dmochowski, J.; Mendola, P.; Sever, L. E.; Fitzgerald, E.; Kostyniak, P.; Greizerstein, H.; and Olson, H. "Parental Consumption of Contaminated Sport Fish from Lake Ontario and Predicted Fecundability." *Epidemiology* 11 (2000): 388–393.

Carter, J. P.; Furman, T.; and Hutcheson, H. R. "Preeclampsia and Reproductive Performance in a Community of Vegans." *Southern Medical Journal* 80 (1987): 692–697.

Clapp, J. F. "Exercise during Pregnancy. A Clinical Update." *Clinical Sports Medicine* 19, no. 2 (2000): 273–286.

Cnattingius, S.; Bergstrom, R.; Lipworth, L.; and Kramer, M. S. "Prepregnancy Weight and the Risk of Adverse Pregnancy Outcomes." *New England Journal of Medicine* 338 (1998): 147–152.

Flaxman, S. M., and Sherman, P. W. "Morning Sickness: A Mechanism for Protecting Mother and Embryo." *Quarterly Review of Biology* 75, no. 2 (2000): 113–148.

Godfrey, K. M., and Barker, D. J. P. "Fetal Nutrition and Adult Disease." *American Journal of Clinical Nutrition* 71 (2000): 1344S–1352S.

Hornstra, G. "Essential Fatty Acids in Mothers and Their Neonates." *American Journal of Clinical Nutrition* 71 (2000): 1262S–1269S.

Jacobson, J. L., and Jacobson, S. W. "Evidence of PCBs as Neurodevelopmental Toxicants in Humans." *Neurotoxicology* 18, no. 2 (1997): 415–424.

Mangels, R. "Vegetarian Diets during Pregnancy." *Issues in Vegetarian Dietetics* 9, no. 1 (1999): 1, 5–8.

Messina, M., and Messina, V. *The Dietitian's Guide to Vegetarian Diets: Issues and Applications.* Gaithersburg, Md.: Aspen, 1996.

Chapter 4: Worry-Free Breastfeeding

Ahlborg, U. G.; Lipworth, L.; Titus-Ernstoff, L.; et al. "Organochlorine Compounds in Relation to Breast Cancer, Endometrial Cancer, and Endometriosis: An Assessment of the Biological and Epidemiological Evidence." *Critical Reviews in Toxicology* 25 (1995): 463–531.

American Academy of Pediatrics Work Group on Breastfeeding. "Breastfeeding and the Use of Human Milk." *Pediatrics* 100, no. 6 (1997): 1035–1039.

American Academy of Pediatrics Work Group on Cow's Milk Protein and Diabetes Mellitus. "Infant Feeding Practices and Their Possible Relationship to the Etiology of Diabetes Mellitus." *Pediatrics* 94 (1994): 752–754.

Clyne, P. S., and Kulczycki, A. "Human Breast Milk Contains Bovine IgG. Relationship to Infant Colic?" *Pediatrics* 87 (1991): 439–444.

Hergenrather, J.; Hlady, G.; Wallace, B.; and Savage, E. "Pollutants in Breast Milk of Vegetarians." *New England Journal of Medicine* 304 (1981): 792.

Koninckx, P. K.; Braet, P.; Kennedy, S. H.; and Barlow, D. H. "Dioxin Pollution and Endometriosis in Belgium." *Human Reproduction* 9 (1994): 1001–1002.

La Leche League, "Advantages of Breastfeeding, Frequently Asked Questions, 1996." http://www.lalecheleague.org/FAQ/FAQadvantage.html

Lust, K. D.; Brown, J. E.; and Thomas, W. "Maternal Intake of Cruciferous Vegetables and Other Foods and Colic Symptoms in Exclusively Breast-fed Infants." *Journal of the American Dietetic Association* 96 (1996): 46–48.

Smith, M. E. "Nursing the World Back to Health." *New Beginnings* 12, no. 3 (1995): 68–71.

Chapter 5: The Transition to Solid Foods

Krebs-Smith, S. M.; Cook, A.; Subar, A. F.; Cleveland, L.; Friday, J.; and Kahle, L. L. "Fruit and Vegetable Intakes of Children and Adolescents in the United States." *Archives of Pediatric and Adolescent Medicine* 150, no. 1 (1996): 81–86.

Webber, L. S.; Dalferes, E. R. Jr.; and Strong, J. P. "Atherosclerosis of the Aorta and Coronary Arteries and Cardiovascular Risk Factors in Persons Aged 6 to 30 Years and Studied at Necropsy (The Bogalusa Heart Study)." *American Journal of Cardiology* 70, no. 9 (1992): 851–858.

Ziegler, E. E.; Fomon, S. J.; Nelson, S. E.; Rebouche, C. J.; Edwards, B. B.; Rogers, R. R.; and Lehman, L. J. "Cow Milk Feeding in Infancy: Further Observations on Blood Loss from the Gastrointestinal Tract." *Journal of Pediatrics* 116 (1990): 11–18.

Chapter 6: Feeding Toddlers

Dennison, B. A.; Rockwell, H. L.; and Baker, S. L. "Excess Fruit Juice Consumption by Preschool-Aged Children Is Associated with Short Stature and Obesity." *Pediatrics* 99 (1997): 15–22.

Messina, M., and Messina, V. *The Dietitian's Guide to Vegetarian Diets: Issues and Applications.* Gaithersburg, Md.: Aspen, 1996.

Chapter 7: Growing Kids

American Academy of Pediatrics Committee on Nutrition. "Statement on Cholesterol." *Pediatrics* 90 (1992): 469–472.

Attwood, C. R. *Dr. Attwood's Low-Fat Prescription for Kids.* New York: Penguin, 1995.

Demas, A. "Low-Fat School Lunch Programs: Achieving Acceptance." *American Journal of Cardiology* 82, no. 10B (1998): 80T–82T.

DISC Collaborative Research Group. "Efficacy and Safety of Lowering Dietary Intake of Fat and Cholesterol in Children with Elevated Low-Density Lipoprotein Cholesterol." *Journal of the American Medical Association* 273 (1995): 1429–1435.

Kimm, S. Y. S.; Gergen, P. J.; Malloy, M.; Dresser, C.; and Carroll, M. "Dietary Patterns of U.S. Children: Implications for Disease Prevention." *Preventive Medicine* 19 (1990): 432–442.

U.S. Department of Agriculture, Agricultural Research Service. 1999. "Food and Nutrient Intakes by Children 1994–1996," 1998. Online ARS Food Surveys Research Group available at http://www.barc.usda.gov/bhnrc/foodsurvey/home.htm (accessed December 18, 2000).

Chapter 8: The Teen Years

Barnard, N. D.; Scialli, A. R.; Hurlock, D.; and Bertron, P. "Diet and Sex-Hormone Binding Globulin, Dysmenorrhea, and Premenstrual Symptoms." *Obstetrics and Gynecology* 95 (2000): 245–250.

Berkey, C. S.; Frazier, A. L.; Gardner, J. D.; et al. "Adolescence and Breast Carcinoma Risk." *Cancer* 85 (1999): 2400–2409.

Berkey, C. S.; Gardner, J. D.; Frazier, A. L.; and Colditz, G. A. "Relation of Childhood Diet and Body Size to Menarche and Adolescent Growth in Girls." *American Journal of Epidemiology* 152 (2000): 446–462.

Cameron, J. L. "Nutritional Determinants of Puberty." *Nutrition Reviews* II (1996): S17–S22.

Falkner, B.; Sherif, K.; Michel, S.; and Kushner, H. "Dietary Nutrients and Blood Pressure in Urban Minority Adolescents at Risk for Hypertension." *Archives of Pediatric and Adolescent Medicine* 154 (2000): 918–922.

Kahn, L.; Warren, C. W.; Harris, W. A.; Collins, J. L.; Douglas, K. A.; Collins, M. E.; Williams, B. I.; Ross, J. G.; and Koble, L. J. "Youth Risk Behavior Surveillance—United States, 1993." In *CDC Surveillance Summaries,* March 24, 1995. *Morbidity and Mortality Weekly Report* 44, no. SS-1 (1995): 1–56.

Lytle, L. A.; Seifert, S.; Greenstein, J.; and McGovern, P. "How Do Children's Eating Patterns and Food Choices Change over Time? Results from a Cohort Study." *American Journal of Health Promotion* 14, no. 4 (2000): 222–228.

Malina, R. M. "Physical Growth and Biological Maturation of Young Athletes." *Exercise and Sport Sciences Reviews* 22 (1994): 389–433.

Messina, M, and Messina, V. *The Dietitian's Guide to Vegetarian Diets: Issues and Applications.* Gaithersburg, Md.: Aspen, 1996.

Neumark-Sztainer, D.; Story, M.; Resnick, M. D.; and Blum, R. W. "Correlates of Inadequate Fruit and Vegetable Consumption among Adolescents." *Preventive Medicine* 25 (1995): 497–505.

Rogol, A. D.; Clark, P. A.; and Roemmich, J. N. "Growth and Pubertal Development in Children and Adolescents: Effects of Diet and Physical Activity." *American Journal of Clinical Nutrition* 72 (2000): 521S–528S.

Rosner, B.; Colditz, G. A.; and Willett, W. C. "Reproductive Risk Factors in a Prospective Study of Breast Cancer." *American Journal of Epidemiology* 139 (1994): 819–835.

Zheng, W.; Dai, Q.; Custer, L. J.; Shu, X. O.; Wen, W. Q.; Jin, F.; and Franke, A. A. "Urinary Excretion of Isoflavinoids and the Risk of Breast Cancer." *Cancer Epidemiology, Biomarkers and Prevention* 8, no. 1 (1999): 35–40.

Chapter 9: Foods and Common Health Problems

American Academy of Pediatrics Work Group on Cow's Milk Protein and Diabetes Mellitus. "Infant Feeding Practices and Their Possible Relationship to the Etiology of Diabetes Mellitus." *Pediatrics* 94 (1994): 752–754.

Barnard, N. *Eat Right, Live Longer.* New York: Three Rivers Press, 1996.

Carey, O. J.; Cookson, J. B.; Britton, J.; and Tattersfield, A. E. "The Effect of Lifestyle on Wheeze, Atopy, and Bronchial Hyperreactivity in Asian and White Children." *American Journal of Respiratory and Critical Care Medicine* 153 (1996): 537–540.

Cuatrecasas, P.; Lockwood, D. H.; and Caldwell, J. R. "Lactase Deficiency in the Adult: A Common Occurrence." *Lancet* 1 (1965): 14–18.

Daher, S.; Sole, D.; and de Morais, M. B. "Cow's Milk and Chronic Constipation in Children." *New England Journal of Medicine* 340 (1998): 891.

Fogarty, A., and Britton, J. "Nutritional Issues and Asthma." *Current Opinion in Pulmonary Medicine* 6, no. 1 (2000): 86–89.

Hertzler, S. R.; Huynh, B. C. L.; and Savaiano, D. A. "How Much Lactose Is Low Lactose?" *Journal of the American Dietetic Association* 96 (1996): 243–246.

Hijazi, N.; Abalkhail, B.; and Seaton, A. "Diet and Childhood Asthma in a Society in Transition: A Study in Urban and Rural Saudi Arabia." *Thorax* 55, no. 9 (2000): 775–779.

Huang, S. S, and Bayless, T. M. "Milk and Lactose Intolerance in Healthy Orientals." *Science* 160 (1968): 83–84.

Iacono, G.; Cavataio, F.; Montalto, G.; Florena. A.; et al. "Intolerance of Cow's Milk and Chronic Constipation in Children." *New England Journal of Medicine* 339 (1998): 1100–1104.

Juntti, H.; Tikkanen. S.; Kokkonen, J.; Alho, O. P.; and Niinimaki, A. "Cow's Milk Allergy Is Associated with Recurrent Otitis Media during Childhood." *Acta Otolaryngology* 119 (1999): 867–873.

Lindahl, O.; Lindwall, L.; Spangberg, A.; and Ockerman, P. A. "Vegan Regimen with Reduced Medication in the Treatment of Bronchial Asthma." *Journal of Asthma* 22, no. 1 (1985): 45–55.

Mishkin, S. "Dairy Sensitivity, Lactose Malabsorption, and Elimination Diets in Inflammatory Bowel Disease." *American Journal of Clinical Nutrition* 65 (1997): 564–567.

Newcomer, A. D.; Gordon, H.; Thomas, P. J.; and McGill, D. G. "Family Studies of Lactase Deficiency in the American Indian." *Gastroenterology* 73 (1977): 985–988.

Nsouli, T. M.; Nsouli, S. M.; Linde, R. D.; O'Mara, F.; Scanlon, R. T.; and, Bellanti, J. A. "Role of Food Allergy in Serous Otitis Media." *Annals of Allergy* 73 (1994): 215–219.

Shah, N.; Lindley, K.; and Milla, P. "Cow's Milk and Chronic Constipation in Children." *New England Journal of Medicine* 340 (1998): 892.

Sridhar, M. K. "Nutrition and Lung Health." *Proceedings of the Nutrition Society* 58, no. 2 (1999): 303–308.

Woteki, C. E.; Weser, E.; and Young, E. A. "Lactose Malabsorption in Mexican American Adults." *American Journal of Clinical Nutrition* 30 (1977): 470–475.

Yazicioglu, M.; Baspinar, I.; Ones, U.; Pala, O.; and Kiziler, U. "Egg and Milk Allergy in Asthmatic Children: Assessment by Immulite Allergy Food Panel, Skin Prick Tests and Double-Blind Placebo-Controlled Food Challenges." *Allergologia et Immunopathologia* 27, no. 6 (1999): 287–293.

Chapter 10: Feeding the Mind

American Psychiatric Association. *Diagnostic and Statistical Manual of Mental Disorders,* 4th ed. Washington, D.C.: American Psychiatric Association, 1994.

Anderson, J. W.; Johnstone, B. M.; and Remley, D. T. "Breastfeeding and Cognitive Development: A Meta-analysis." *American Journal of Clinical Nutrition* 70 (1999): 525–535.

Bellisle, F.; Blundell, J.; Dye, L.; Fantino, M.; Fern, E.; Fletcher, R. J.; Lambert, J.; Roberfroid, M.; Specter, S.; Westenhofer, J.; and Westerterp-Plantenga, M. S. "Functional Food Science and Behaviour and Psychological Function." *British Journal of Nutrition* 80 (1998): 173S–193S.

Kaplan, B. J.; McNicol, J.; Conte, R. A.; and Moghadam, H. K. "Dietary Replacement in Preschool-Aged Hyperactive Boys." *Pediatrics* 83, no. 1 (1989): 7–17.

Knivsberg, A.; Wiig, K.; Lind, G.; Nodland, M.; and Reichelt, K. "Dietary Intervention in Autistic Syndromes." *Brain Dysfunction* 3 (1990): 315–327.

Lucarelli, S.; Frediani, T.; Zingoni, A. M.; Ferruzzi, F.; Giardini, O.; Quintieri, F.; Barbato, M.; D'Eufemia, P.; and Cardi, E. "Food Allergy and Infantile Autism." *Panminerva Medica* 37, no. 3 (1995): 137–141.

Pollitt, E. "Does Breakfast Make a Difference in School?" *Journal of the American Dietetic Association* 95 (1995): 1134–1139.

Statement of the Standing Committee on Nutrition of the British Paediatric Association. "Is Breastfeeding Beneficial in the U.K.?" *Archives of Disease in Childhood* 72 (1994): 376–380.

Chapter 11: Healthy Eating for the Young Athlete

Berning, J., and Steen, S. N. *The School-Aged Child Athlete: Nutrition for Sport and Exercise.* Gaithersburg, Md.: Aspen, 1997.

Lanou, A. *The Pathway to Better Health.* Ithaca, N.Y.: New Century Nutrition, 1996.

Chapter 12: Nurturing a Healthy Body Image

Cooke, K. *Real Gorgeous: The Truth about Body & Beauty.* New York: W. W. Norton, 1996.

Chapter 13: Achieving a Healthy Weight and Fitness Level

Attwood, C. R. *Dr. Attwood's Low-Fat Prescription for Kids.* New York: Penguin Books, 1995.

Birch, L. L., and Fisher, J. O. "Mothers' Child Feeding Practices Influence Daughters' Eating and Weight." *American Journal of Clinical Nutrition* 71 (2000): 1054–1061.

Centers for Disease Control and Prevention. *CDC Surveillance Summaries, July 7, 2000. Morbidity and Mortality Weekly Report* 49, no. SS-6 (2000): 1–39.

Dywer, J. T.; Stone, E. J.; Yang, M.; Webber, L. S.; Must, A.; Feldman, H. A.; Nader, P. R.; Perry, C. L.; and Parcel, G. S. "Prevalence of Marked Overweight and Obesity in a Multiethnic Pediatric Population: Findings from the Child and Adolescent Trial for Cardiovascular Health (CATCH) Study." *Journal of the American Dietetic Association* 100, no. 10 (2000): 1149–1156.

Esselstyn, C. B.; Ellis, S. T.; Medendorp, S. V.; and Crowe, T. D. "A Strategy to Arrest and Reverse Coronary Artery Disease: A 5-Year Longitudinal Study of a Single Physician's Practice." *Journal of Family Practice* 41 (1995): 560–568.

Flatt, J. P. McCollum Award Lecture, 1995. "Diet, Lifestyle, and Weight Maintenance." *American Journal of Clinical Nutrition* 62 (1995): 820–836.

Hill, J. O.; Drougas, H.; and Peters, J. C. "Obesity Treatment: Can Diet Composition Play a Role?" *Annals of Internal Medicine* 119 (1993): 694–697.

Hulman, S.; Kushner, H.; Katz, S.; and Falkner, B. "Can Cardiovascular Risk Be Predicted by Newborn, Childhood, and Adolescent Body Size? An Examination of Longitudinal Data in Urban African Americans." *Journal of Pediatrics* 132, no. 1 (1998): 90–97.

Kendall, A.; Levitsky, D. A.; Strupp, B. J.; and Lissner, L. "Weight Loss on a Low-Fat Diet: Consequence of the Imprecision of the Control of Food Intake in Humans." *American Journal of Clinical Nutrition.* 53, no. 5 (1991): 1124–1129.

Melby, C. I.; Goldflies, D. G.; Hyner, G. C. I.; and Lyle, R. M. "Relations between Vegetarian/Nonvegetarian Diets and Blood Pressure in Black and White Adults." *American Journal of Public Health* 79 (1989): 1283–1288.

Must, A.; Jacques, P. F.; Dallal, G. E.; Bajema, C. J.; and Dietz, W. H. "Long-Term Morbidity and Mortality of Overweight Adolescents: A Follow-up of the Harvard Growth Study of 1922 to 1935." *New England Journal of Medicine* 327, no. 19 (1992): 1350–1355.

Neumark-Stainzer, D., and Hannan, P. J. "Weight-Related Behaviors among Adolescent Girls and Boys: Results from a National Survey." *Archives of Pediatric and Adolescent Medicine* 154, no. 6 (2000): 569–577.

Neumark-Stainzer, D.; Rock, C. L.; Thornquist, M. D.; Cheskin, L. J.; Neuhouser, M. L.; and Barnett, M. J. "Weight-Control Behaviors among

Adults and Adolescents: Associations with Dietary Intake." *Preventive Medicine* 30, no. 5 (2000): 381–391.

Ogden, C. L.; Troiano, R. P.; Briefel, R. R.; Kuczmarski, R. J.; Flegal, K. M.; and Johnson, C. L. "Prevalence of Overweight among Preschool Children in the United States, 1971 through 1994." *Pediatrics* 99, no. 4 (1997): E1.

Ornish, D.; Scherwitz, L. W.; Billings, J. H.; Brown, S. E.; Gould, K. L.; Merritt, T. A.; Sparler, S.; Armstrong, W. T.; Ports, T. A.; Kirkeeide, R. L.; Hogeboom, C.; and Brand, R. J. "Intensive Lifestyle Changes for Reversal of Coronary Heart Disease." *Journal of the American Medical Association* 280, no. 23 (1998): 2001–2007.

Shintani, T. T.; Hughes, C. K.; Beckham, S.; and O'Connor, H. K. "Obesity and Cardiovascular Risk Intervention through the Ad Libitum Feeding of Traditional Hawaiian Diet." *American Journal of Clinical Nutrition* 53 (1991): 1647S–1651S.

Snowdon, D. A., and Phillips, R. L. "Does a Vegetarian Diet Reduce the Occurrence of Diabetes?" *American Journal of Public Health* 75 (1985): 507–512.

Spock, B., and Parker, S. J. *Dr. Spock's Baby and Child Care,* 7th ed. New York: Simon & Schuster, 1998.

Vanhalla, M. "Childhood Weight and Metabolic Syndrome in Adults." *Annals of Medicine* 31 (1999): 236–239.

Chapter 14: Eating Disorders: A Guide for Parents

Kaneko, K.; Kiriike, N.; Ikenaga, K.; Miyawaki, D. M.; and Yamagami, S. "Weight and Shape Concerns and Dieting Behaviours among Preadolescents and Adolescents in Japan." *Psychiarty and Clinical Neurosciences* 53, no. 3 (1999): 365–371.

Lee, S., and Lee, A. M. "Disordered Eating in Three Communities of China: A Comparative Study of Female High School Students in Hong Kong, Shenzhen, and Rural Hunan." *International Journal of Eating Disorders* 27, no. 3 (2000): 317–327.

Martin, A. R.; Nieto, J. M.; Jimenez, M. A.; Ruiz, J. P.; Vazquez, M. C.; Fernandez, Y. C.; Gomex, M. A.; and Fernandez, C. C. "Unhealthy Eating Behaviour in Adolescents." *European Journal of Epidemiology* 15, no. 7 (1999): 643–648.

National Association of Anorexia Nervosa and Associated Disorders. "The High School Study, 1990." http://www.anad.org

Index

Note: An Index of Recipe Titles can be found on pages x–xi.

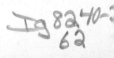